# Spine

*Rehabilitation Medicine Quick Reference*

**Ralph M. Buschbacher, MD**
*Series Editor*

Professor, Department of Physical Medicine and Rehabilitation
Indiana University School of Medicine
Indianapolis, Indiana

## Spine

André Panagos

## Spinal Cord Injury

Thomas N. Bryce

***Forthcoming Volumes in the Series***

Traumatic Brain Injury

Musculoskeletal, Sports, and Occupational Medicine

Pediatrics

Neuromuscular/EMG

Prosthetics

Stroke

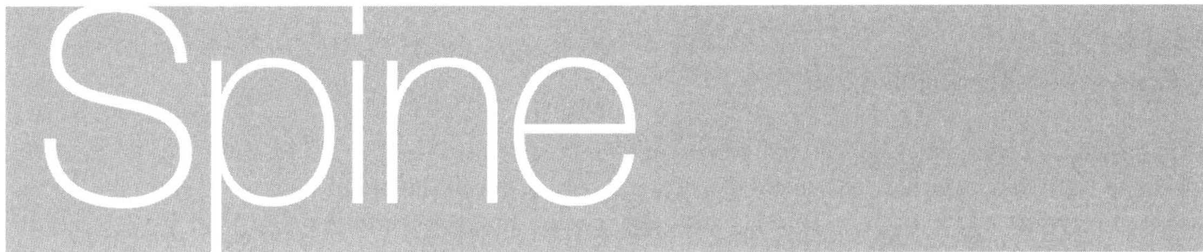


Rehabilitation Medicine Quick Reference

**André Panagos, MD**
Department of Rehabilitation Medicine
New York-Presbyterian Hospital
Weill Cornell Medical Center
New York, New York

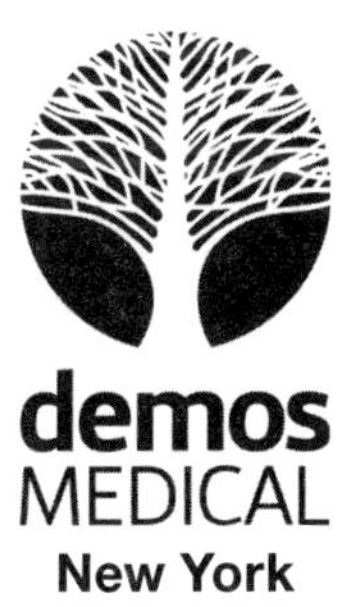

demos
MEDICAL
New York

Acquisitions Editor: Beth Barry
Cover Design: Steve Pisano
Compositor: NewGen North America
Printer: Bang Printing
Visit our website at www.demosmedpub.com





Library of Congress Cataloging-in-Publication Data

Panagos, Andre.
Spine / Andre Panagos.
p. ; cm.—(Rehabilitation medicine quick reference)
Includes bibliographical references and index.
ISBN 978-1-933864-28-0 (alk. paper)
1. Spine—Diseases—Handbooks, manuals, etc. I. Title. II. Series: Rehabilitation medicine quick reference.
[DNLM: 1. Spinal Diseases—Handbooks. 2. Spine—physiopathology—Handbooks. WE 39 P187s 2009]
RD768.P26 2009
616.7′3—dc22 2009022795

Special discounts on bulk quantities of Demos Medical Publishing books are available to corporations, professional associations, pharmaceutical companies, health care organizations, and other qualifying groups. For details, please contact:

Special Sales Department
Demos Medical Publishing
11 West 42nd Street, 15th Floor
New York, NY 10036
Phone: 800-532-8663 or 212-683-0072
Fax: 212-941-7842
Email: orderdept@demosmedpub.com

Made in the United States of America

09 10 11 12 5 4 3 2 1

*To my wife, Sophia,*

*whose love and unwavering support enriched each page,*

*and to our daughter, Marilia,*

*who blessed us with her birth during this project.*

# Contents

# List of Acronyms

| | |
|---|---|
| CSF | cerebrospinal fluid |
| CT | computed tomography |
| MRI | magnetic resonance imaging |
| NSAID | nonsteroidal anti-inflammatory drugs |
| PET | positron emission tomography |
| RA | rheumatoid arthritis |
| SCI | spinal cord injury |
| SPECT | single-photon emission computed tomography |

# Series Foreword

The Rehabilitation Medicine Quick Reference (RMQR) series is dedicated to the busy clinician. While we all strive to keep up with the latest medical knowledge, there are many times when things come up in our daily practices that we need to look up. Even more importantly . . . look up quickly.

Those aren't the times to do a complete literature search or to read a detailed chapter or review article. We just need to get a quick grasp of a topic that we may not see routinely, or just to refresh our memory. Sometimes a subject comes up that is outside our usual scope of practice, but that may still impact our care. It is for such moments that this series has been created.

Whether you need to quickly look up what a Tarlov cyst is, or you need to read about a neurorehabilitation complication or treatment, RMQR has you covered.

RMQR is designed to include the most common problems found in a busy practice, but also a lot of the less common ones as well.

I was extremely lucky to have been able to assemble an absolutely fantastic group of editors. They in turn have harnessed an excellent set of authors. So what we have in this series is, I hope and believe, a tremendous reference set to be used often in daily clinical practice. As series editor, I have of course been privy to these books before actual publication. I can tell you that I have already started to rely on them in my clinic—often. They have helped me become more efficient in practice.

Each chapter is organized into succinct facts, presented in a bullet point style. The chapters are set up in the same way throughout all of the volumes in the series, so once you get used to the format, it is incredibly easy to look things up.

And while the focus of the RMQR series is, of course, rehabilitation medicine, the clinical applications are much broader.

I hope that each reader grows to appreciate the Rehabilitation Medicine Quick Reference series as much as I have. I congratulate a fine group of editors and authors on creating readable and useful texts.

**Ralph M. Buschbacher, MD**

# Preface

This book was conceived as a quick reference guide for the most common spine disorders. It was born out of my frustration in finding relevant research articles to help in evaluating and treating complex patients that I saw in our spine center. For many conditions, relevant information was difficult to find and the law of parsimony was of limited value.

This text is broken down into the 100 most common spine disorders, with each topic presented in a clear and consistent two-page format. There were a larger number of etiologies that I uncovered, but in many cases there was little scientific literature available. Finding research literature on the conditions that I did include was also sometimes challenging. I also took the liberty to include a section on common spine-mimicking conditions as they are sometimes indistinguishable from true spine disorders.

This book would not have been possible had it not been for my mentors in physical medicine and rehabilitation who provided the mandate and led the way in spine care: Stanley Herring, MD, Stuart Kahn, MD, and Willibald Nagler, MD. I would also like to acknowledge Michael W. O'Dell, MD, who supported my intellectual motivation to tackle this project; and acknowledge my collegues, Roger Hartl, MD, Keith Hentel, MD, Matthew Lipp, MD, and Tracy Maltz, DPT, who always challenge me with new and interesting cases. Finally, I would like to thank our residents and visiting medical students who were courageous enough to ask the questions that only raw curiosity puts forth.

There were, of course, triumphs and failures as I compiled the "Top 100" and I hope that through my frustration I have improved your outcomes in the battlefield of spine care.

**André Panagos, MD**

# Spine

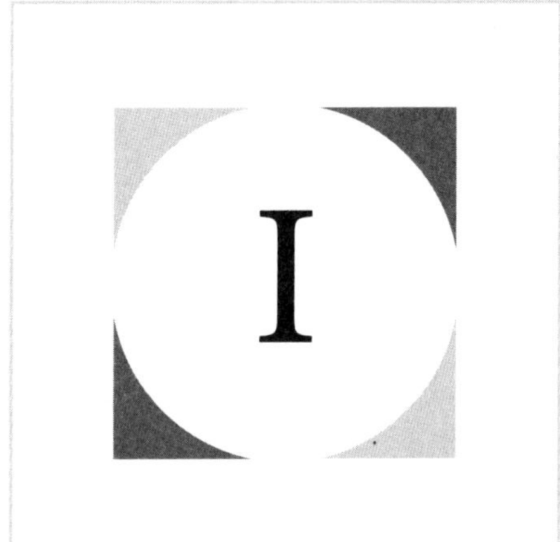

# Conditions of the Spine

# Achondroplasia

## Description

Achondroplasia is the most common form of dwarfism, resulting in a characteristically large head with frontal bossing and a long narrow trunk with short limbs.

## Etiology/Types

- Autosomal-dominant inheritance
- Fibroblast growth factor receptor 3 (*FGFR3*) gene point mutation causes 95% of cases.
- 80% of cases are new mutations.

## Epidemiology

- Achondroplasia is the most common form of dwarfism.
- Occurs in 1 in 10,000 to 30,000 live births
- Affects 250,000 individuals worldwide

## Pathogenesis

- Decreased endochondral bone growth

## Risk Factors

- Familial inheritance
- Spontaneous mutation risk factors are unknown.

## Clinical Features

- Large head with frontal bossing
- Hypoplastic midface
- Long narrow trunk with short limbs
- Joint hyperextensibility affecting the hands and knees
- Restricted elbow rotation and extension
- Thoracolumbar gibbus may develop by 4 months of age leading to a fixed kyphoscoliosis.
- Exaggerated lumbar lordosis
- Infants may develop respiratory distress due to cervical medullary compression.
- Motor development may be delayed due to narrowing of the foramen magnum.
- Tibial bowing affects 42% of the population.
- Neurogenic claudication and spinal stenosis are common in older children and adults.

## Natural History

- Cervical and lumbar spinal stenosis with aging
- Increasing back pain due to spinal stenosis, exaggerated lumbar lordosis, and spondylosis
- 10% of affected individuals have neurogenic claudication by 10 years of age.
- 80% of affected individuals have neurogenic claudication by 60 years of age.

## Diagnosis

### *Differential diagnosis*

- Hypochondroplasia
- Severe achondroplasia with developmental delay and acanthosis nigricans
- Thanatophoric dysplasia types I and II

### *History*

- Increasing neck or low back pain
- Increased weakness
- Decreased function and mobility

### *Exam*

- Short stature
- Large head with frontal bossing
- Hypoplastic midface
- Long narrow trunk with short limbs
- Lower motor neuron or upper motor neuron findings
- Fixed kyphoscoliosis or exaggerated lumbar lordosis

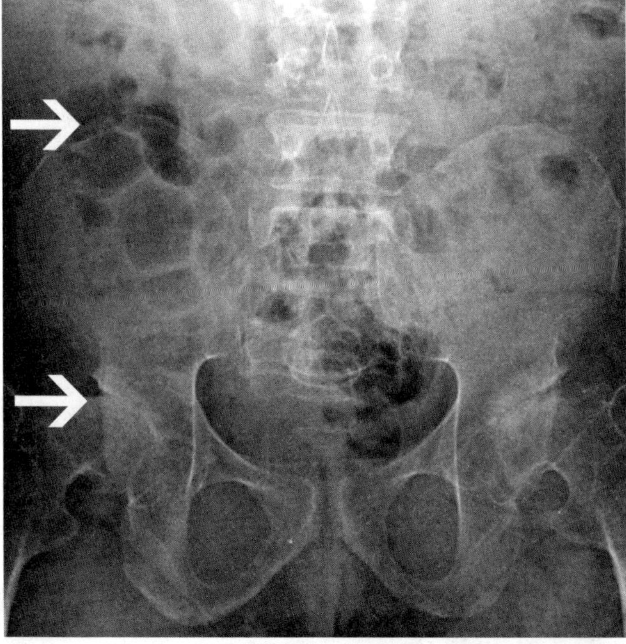

Anteriopostèrior pelvis plain radiograph demonstrating narrowed and relatively higher iliac wings and flattened acetabulae with short femoral necks. (Courtesy of Keith Hentel, MD.)

### Testing

- DNA testing
- X-rays demonstrate normal height and width of vertebral bodies with short, thickened pedicles throughout the spine.
- Narrowed central spinal canal
- Exaggerated lumbar lordosis
- Computed tomography (CT) is used to assess for medullary compression due to craniocervical stenosis.
- Somatosensory evoked potentials (SSEP) may be used to assess cervical cord compression.
- Electrodiagnostic studies to assess radicular symptoms

### Pitfalls

- Repetitive nerve compression injuries may result in irreversible muscle atrophy and loss of mobility.

## Red flags

- Tetraplegia
- Cauda equina syndrome

## Treatment

### Medical

- Nonsteroidal anti-inflammatory drugs (NSAIDs)
- A trial of bracing may be helpful for back pain and curvature reduction.

### Exercises

- General strengthening and stretching

### Modalities

- Heat, cold, ultrasound, and transcutaneous electrical nerve stimulation have been used for symptomatic relief of pain and muscle spasms.

### Injection

- Trigger point injections for symptoms of myofascial pain
- Epidural steroid injection for radicular symptoms

### Surgical

- 5% to 10% of patients have cervical medullary decompression surgery as early as infancy.
- Extensive decompressive laminectomy may need to be performed, which may involve the entire spine.
- Reoperation may be required within 8 years.

### Consults

- Physical medicine and rehabilitation
- Neurologic or orthopedic-spine surgery
- Neurology

### Complications of treatment

- Syringomyelia
- Tetraplegia
- Persistent and severe sciatica
- Cauda equina syndrome

## Prognosis

- Continued function is possible if assessed early and surgically treated.

## Helpful Hints

- Repetitive nerve compression injuries may result in irreversible muscle atrophy and loss of mobility, so early treatment is important.

## Suggested Readings

Horton WA, Hall JG, Hecht JT. Achondroplasia. *Lancet.* 2007;370(9582):162–172.

Siebens AA, Hungerford DS, Kirby NA. Achondroplasia: effectiveness of an orthosis in reducing deformity of the spine. *Arch Phys Med Rehabil.* 1987;68(6):384–388.

# Aging Lumbosacral Spine

## Description

With aging, the initial intervertebral disc degeneration is followed by progressive deterioration of the adjacent bone, muscles, zygapophyseal (facet) joints, and ligaments.

## Etiology/Types

- Difficult to differentiate normal aging from pathologic processes
- Genetic inheritance accounts for 50% to 70% of disc degeneration variability.
- High or repetitive mechanical loading and smoking are thought to play a role.

## Epidemiology

- Universal
- Progression varies widely.

## Pathogenesis

- The anterior column carries 75% of the total axial compressive load.
- The intervertebral disc can withstand 2.8 to 13.0 kN of compressive force.
- Intradiscal proteoglycan content progressively declines with advancing age.
- Vertebral endplate permeability decreases beginning in the second decade of life.
- Changes first affect the endplate, followed by the nucleus pulposus and the annulus fibrosis over several spinal levels.
- Calcified nucleus pulposus herniation through the endplate is called a Schmorl's node.
- Degeneration of the normally avascular intervertebral disc allows blood vessels and nociceptive fibers to penetrate the disc, introducing inflammatory mediators into the previously avascular space.
- The degenerative cascade describes the loss of hydrostatic pressure within the nucleus pulposus, resulting in increased compressive loads on the annulus fibrosis and zygapophyseal (facet) joints.
- Intervertebral disc injuries never fully heal.
- Osteophytes increase the load-bearing surface area.
- The aging ligamentum flavum loses elastin content, causing anterior bulging that can contribute to central spinal stenosis.
- Loss of dorsal extensor muscle and the abdominal flexors muscle equilibrium

## Risk Factors

- Genetic inheritance
- High or repetitive mechanical loading
- Smoking

## Clinical Features

- Ranges from painless progression to severe back pain
- Progressive weakness
- Loss of flexibility

## Natural History

- Narrowing in adult intervertebral discs occurs at a rate of 3% per year.
- The majority of acute disc herniations occur between the ages of 30 and 50.
- 90% of lumbar discs demonstrate degeneration by the fifth decade of life.

## Diagnosis

### *Differential diagnosis*

- Fracture
- Infection
- Neoplasm
- Stenosis

### *History*

- Deep dull lumbosacral ache
- Radiation into the buttock or posterior thighs
- Morning stiffness

### *Exam*

- Lumbosacral paraspinal tenderness
- Pelvic girdle muscle atrophy

### *Testing*

- X-rays demonstrate degenerative changes in 90% of patients.
- Magnetic resonance imaging (MRI) can identify disc degeneration in 35% of healthy volunteers.
- Larger disc herniations seen on initial imaging correspond with greater resolution of the herniation in 2 years.
- No correlation with pain and disc signal intensity on MRI

### *Pitfalls*

- Overinterpretation of imaging findings

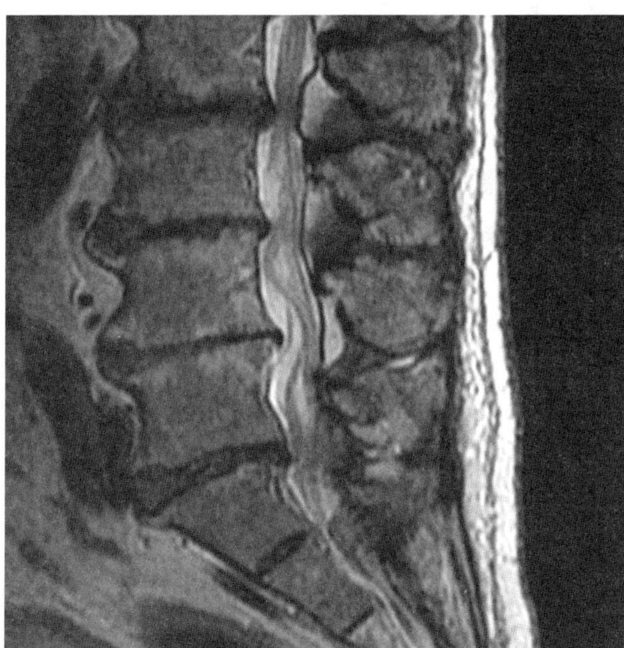

Sagittal lumbar T2-weighted magnetic resonance image demonstrating multilevel disc degeneration that is often associated with aging.

## Red Flags

- Fracture
- Infection
- Neoplasm
- Neurologic dysfunction

## Treatment

### *Medical*

- NSAIDs
- Analgesics
- Acupuncture has been described as helpful.

### *Exercises*

- Lumbar stabilization focuses on stabilizing the painful pathologic region with muscular development and movement patterns.
- Flexion or extension bias in stretching and strengthening
- Mechanical evaluation to determine a direction of preference

### *Modalities*

- Heat, cold, ultrasound, and transcutaneous electrical nerve stimulation have been used for symptomatic relief of pain and muscle spasms.

### *Injection*

- Trigger point injections for symptoms of myofascial pain
- Epidural steroid injections for symptoms related to radiculitis, radiculopathy, or stenosis

### *Surgical*

- Decompression
- Fusion for unrelenting pain

### *Consults*

- Physical medicine and rehabilitation
- Neurologic or orthopedic-spine surgery

### *Complications of treatment*

- Progressive pain and dysfunction even with appropriate treatment

## Prognosis

- Highly variable

## Helpful Hints

- Disc degeneration is an irreversible process in which intact tissue is unable to respond to progressive structural failures.

## Suggested Readings

Benoist M. Natural history of the aging spine. *Eur Spine J.* 2003;12(Suppl 2):S86–S89.

Kirkaldy-Willis WH, Wedge JH, Yong-Hing K, Reilly J. Pathology and pathogenesis of lumbar spondylosis and stenosis. *Spine.* 1978;3(4):319–328.

# Aneurysmal Bone Cysts

## Description

Aneurysmal bone cysts are benign cystic hyperemic/hemorrhagic lesions.

## Etiology/Types

Thought to be caused by trauma, which allows blood to pool within the bone, resulting in increased intraosseous pressure followed by resorption and cyst formation.

## Epidemiology

- Represents 1% or 2% of all primary bone lesions
- Represents 15% of all primary spine tumors
- 10% to 30% occur in the spine, and the remainder occur in the long bones.
- Primarily occurs in young adults who are under 30 years of age.
- 50% of patients are pediatric.
- Females slightly more affected than males

## Pathogenesis

- Cystic structure with vascular channels of unclotted blood
- May contain immature bony trabeculae, fibrous connective tissue, osteoid, multinucleated giant cells, and granulation tissue.
- Most commonly found in the posterior elements followed by the vertebral body.

## Risk Factors

- Trauma

## Clinical Features

- Acute localized pain and swelling
- Duration of pain may be from months to several years.
- Severity is associated with location and may include sensory changes, paraplegia, neuropathy, or cauda equina syndrome.

## Natural History

- Pain for several months to years
- Increased risk for pathologic bone fractures

## Diagnosis

### *Differential diagnosis*

- Chondroblastoma
- Giant cell tumor
- Infection
- Metastasis

### *History*

- Acute localized pain and swelling

### *Exam*

- Tenderness to local palpation
- Associated muscle spasm
- Decreased range of motion
- Kyphosis or scoliosis

### *Testing*

- X-rays demonstrate a solitary osteolytic lesion with a subperiosteal shell of bone.
- MRI can delineate soft tissue expansion and detect a fluid level on T2-weighted sequences.
- CT scan may show multiple-fluid levels with a thin rim of bone.
- Biopsy

### *Pitfalls*

- Sacral lesions are associated with increased pathologic fractures, and a higher recurrence rate.

## Red Flags

- Cauda equina syndrome
- Neuropathy
- Paraplegia

## Treatment

### *Medical*

- Analgesics

### *Exercises*

- None

### *Modalities*

- None

### *Injection*

- None

### *Surgical*

- Preoperative arterial embolization
- En bloc resection is the preferred treatment, as there is no risk of local recurrence.
- Posterior element involvement may be treated with resection and bone graft.

- Radiotherapy is preferred for large lesions.
- Cryosurgery may halt expansion and prevent recurrence.

### *Consults*

- Neurologic or orthopedic-spine surgery
- Radiation oncology

### *Complications of treatment*

- High intraoperative and postoperative morbidity

## Prognosis

- Commonly recur after curettage
- Early detection and treatment allows for an improved prognosis
- The location of the tumor affects the prognosis
- The maximum rate of local recurrence is one year
- Irradiated patients should be followed for a lifetime due to the small risk of malignant transformation.

## Helpful Hints

- Early diagnosis and treatment leads to a good prognosis and minimal morbidity.

## Suggested Readings

Boriani S, De Iure F, Campanacci L, et al. Aneurysmal bone cyst of the mobile spine: report on 41 cases. *Spine.* 2001;26(1):27–35.

Papagelopoulos PJ, Currier BL, Shaughnessy WJ, et al. Aneurysmal bone cyst of the spine. Management and outcome. *Spine.* 1998;23(5):621–628.

# Ankylosing Spondylitis

## Description

Ankylosing spondylitis is a chronic inflammatory disease that involves the joints of the axial spine and the sacroiliac joint.

## Etiology/Types

- Unknown

## Epidemiology

- Prevalence between 0.1% and 1.4%
- Male to female ratio of 2:1
- Most common in males 15 to 40 years of age

## Pathogenesis

- Thought to be caused by infection, trauma, or heredity

## Risk Factors

- HLA-B27 association
- A positive family history increases the risk up to 30% in HLA-B27–positive first-degree relatives.

## Clinical Features

- Lower back pain is worse in the morning or with inactivity and improves with exercise.
- Lumbosacral back pain occurs in 81% of patients.
- Pseudosciatica due to piriformis muscle spasm and sciatic nerve compression
- Neck stiffness, pain, or torticollis
- 13% of patients develop peripheral joint involvement, acute iridocyclitis, plantar fascial enthesis, or Achilles tendonitis.
- 30% of patients may have involvement of the shoulders, elbows, hips, knees, and ankles.

## Natural History

- Osteoproliferation
- Bone and cartilage interface chondritis or osteitis
- Vertebral body erosion due to inflammatory granulation tissue resulting in ankylosis of the joints and ossification of the surrounding ligaments (syndesmophytes)
- Progressive stiffness

## Diagnosis

### *Differential diagnosis*

- Fibromyalgia
- Herniated intervertebral disc
- Infection
- Osteoarthritis
- Other spondyloarthropathies
- Rheumatoid arthritis
- Tumor

### *History*

- Lumbosacral back pain
- Subjective feeling of "stiffness"
- Lower extremity radiation
- Neck stiffness or pain
- Peripheral joint pain

### *Exam*

- Decreased lumbosacral range of motion can be assessed using distance from fingers to the floor or Schober's test.
- Sacroiliac joint provocative maneuvers include FABER, Gaenslen, and Yoeman tests.
- Flattening of the lumbar spine with loss of lumbar lordosis
- Rigid gait

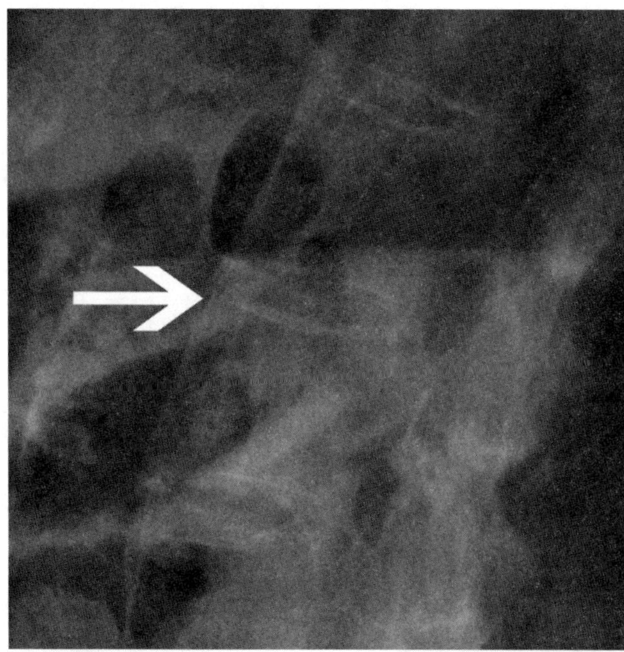

Lateral lumbar plain radiograph in ankylosing spondylitis demonstrating ossification of the anterior longitudinal ligament (arrow) also known as a "bamboo spine." (Adapted from Fast A, Goldsher D. *Navigating the Adult Spine: Bridging Clinical Practice and Neuroradiology.* New York: Demos Medical Publishing, 2007:80.)

### Testing

- 90% of patients are positive for HLA-B27.
- 80% of patients with active disease have an elevated erythrocyte sedimentation rate (ESR).
- X-rays demonstrate bony changes in the sacroiliac joints and loss of the normal lumbar concave surface referred to as a "squared" look.
- Extensive syndesmophyte formation referred to as "bamboo spine"
- MRI localizes early spondylitic changes and contrast enhancement detects early inflammatory lesions within the lumbar spine and sacroiliac joints.

### Pitfalls

- Delayed diagnosis

## Red Flags

- Acute iridocyclitis
- Cauda equina syndrome
- Spinal instability
- Spondylodiscitis

## Treatment

### Medical

- Patient education
- Hard mattress with no pillows for sleeping
- NSAIDs for use in mild to more advanced disease
- Intravenous steroids
- Disease modifying antirheumatic medications for peripheral joint involvement

### Exercises

- Proper posture
- Structured exercise programs have minimal evidence supporting their effectiveness, although they are commonly used.
- Physical therapy should not be too aggressive.
- Strengthening of the extensors of the hip, shoulder, and spine
- Unsupervised exercise for 30 minutes per day, 5 days per week
- General cardiovascular conditioning

### Modalities

- Heat, cold, ultrasound, and transcutaneous electrical nerve stimulation have been used for symptomatic relief of pain and muscle spasms.

### Injection

- None

### Surgical

- Fusion for spinal instability
- Total joint replacements

### Consults

- Physical medicine and rehabilitation
- Neurologic or orthopedic-spine surgery for spinal deformities
- Ophthalmology
- Cardiology for aortic incompetence and conduction deficits
- Pulmonary for fibrotic changes

### Complications of treatment

- Osteoporosis
- Spondylodiscitis

## Prognosis

- Most patients remain functional and employed.
- Worse prognosis with younger age at onset, peripheral joint disease, elevated ESR, and poor response to NSAIDs.

## Helpful Hints

- Pain relief and maintenance of function are the primary treatment goals.

## Suggested Reading

Braun J, Sieper J. Ankylosing spondylitis. *Lancet.* 2007;369(9570):1379–1390.

# Anterior Cord Syndrome (Anterior Spinal Artery Syndrome)

## Description

Anterior cord syndrome is a spinal cord injury characterized by lower extremity paresis or paralysis, loss of pain and temperature sensation below the level of the lesion with preservation of vibratory sense, proprioception, light touch and two-point discrimination.

## Etiology/Types

- Caused by an occlusion of the anterior spinal artery, which supplies blood to the anterior horn and anterior portion of the lateral columns at each level
- Most commonly due to traumatic or ischemic injury to the artery of Adamkiewicz

## Epidemiology

- Comprises 2.7% of all traumatic spinal cord injuries

## Pathogenesis

- The spinal cord is supplied by one anterior and two posterior spinal arteries, which are supplied by radicular arteries that enter the canal through the intervertebral foramen.
- Central arteries originate off of the anterior spinal artery supplying the anterior horn and anterior portion of the lateral columns at each level. The pial plexus surrounding the spinal cord also interconnects the anterior and posterior spinal arteries.
- The C1 to T3 region is perfused by the vertebral arteries at the C3 level and the cervical ascending arteries at the C6–C7 level.
- The T3 to T7 region is perfused by an intercostal artery at the T7 level.
- The T8 to the conus medullaris region is perfused from a branch of the intercostal artery (artery of Adamkiewicz) located between the T9 and T12 levels.

## Risk Factors

- Aortic surgery
- Arterial emboli
- Atherosclerotic narrowing
- Coronary artery bypass graft surgery
- Hypoxemia
- Retroperitoneal dissection
- Thoracic epidural anesthesia

## Clinical Features

- Symptom onset can be rapid, from 2 minutes to several hours.
- Intractable back pain at level of spinal cord ischemia
- Spinothalamic sensory deficits (loss of pain and temperature sensation)
- Preservation of light touch
- Bowel and bladder dysfunction
- Possible respiratory failure

## Natural History

- Rapid development of symptoms, from 2 minutes to several hours

## Diagnosis

### *Differential diagnosis*

- Epidural abscess
- Epidural hematoma

### *History*

- Intractable back pain at the level of spinal cord ischemia
- Bowel and bladder dysfunction
- Motor and sensory deficits

### *Exam*

- Loss of pain and temperature sensation
- Lower extremity paresis or paralysis

### *Testing*

- MRI notes increased T2-weighted signal at the region of the ischemic lesion.

### *Pitfalls*

- Can occur during surgery, allowing the condition to go unnoticed while the patient is anesthetized.

## Red Flags

- Intractable pain
- Lower extremity paresis or paralysis
- Bowel and bladder dysfunction

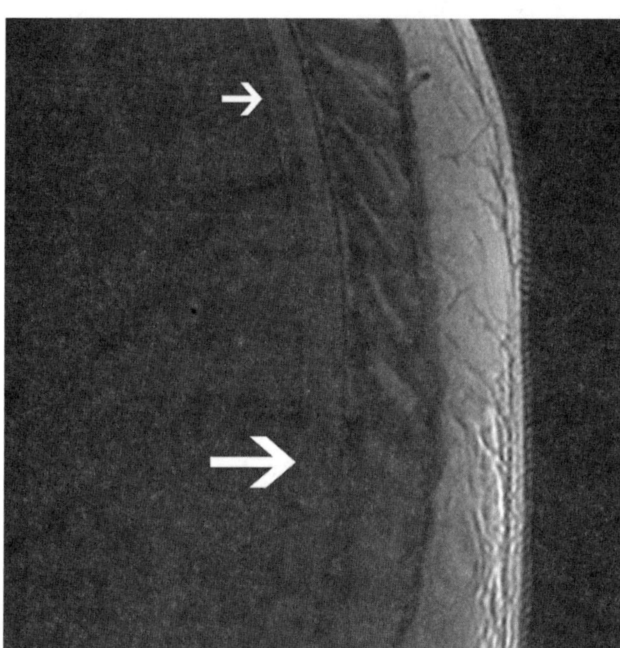

Sagittal thoracic T2-weighted magnetic resonance image demonstrating increased heterogeneous cord signal (arrow), compared to the upper cord that resulted in anterior cord syndrome. (Adapted from Fast A, Goldsher D. *Navigating the Adult Spine: Bridging Clinical Practice and Neuroradiology.* New York: Demos Medical Publishing, 2007:127.)

## Treatment

### Medical

- Vasopressors spare the cerebral and spinal vasculature

### Exercises

- Strengthening and stretching
- Household and community mobility training
- Activities of daily living training

### Modalities

- Heat, cold, ultrasound, and transcutaneous electrical nerve stimulation have been used for symptomatic relief of pain and muscle spasms.

### Injection

- None

### Surgical

- None

### Consults

- Physical medicine and rehabilitation
- Neurology

### Complications of treatment

- Neuropathic pain
- Continued spinal cord injury–related issues

## Prognosis

- Back pain may resolve within days.
- Long-term prognosis is determined by the sparing of the conus medullaris.
- 88% of patients have been successfully discharged home after inpatient rehabilitation.

## Helpful Hints

- Often no identifiable cause can be found.

## Suggested Reading

Baba H, Tomita K, Kawagishi T, Imura S. Anterior spinal artery syndrome. *Int Orthop.* 1993;17(6):353–356.

# Arachnoiditis

## Description

Arachnoiditis is an inflammatory process resulting in fibrosis of the arachnoid membrane causing adherence and entrapment of the adjacent nerve roots.

## Etiology/Types

- Progressive inflammatory reaction
- Possible genetic component resulting in a fibrinolytic defect

## Epidemiology

- Affects up to 11% of failed back surgery syndrome patients

## Pathogenesis

- Following injury, phagocytes and fibrolytic enzymes that usually break down fibrous bands are washed away by the cerebrospinal fluid (CSF).
- Fibrocytes invade the fibrous bands and lay down collagen-forming adhesions around the nerve roots.
- Eventual encapsulation of the nerve roots over several years results in hypoxia and progressive atrophy.

## Risk Factors

- Infection
- Intrathecal depomedrol
- Intrathecal hemorrhage
- Intrathecal medications or anesthetic agents
- Oil- or water-based intrathecal contrast agents
- Retained surgical debris or foreign bodies
- Spinal trauma
- Surgery

## Clinical Features

- Very variable
- Constant neck or back pain
- Pain worsened with activity
- Radicular symptoms
- Bladder dysfunction

## Natural History

- Constant pain with limited function
- Symptoms usually do not progress.

## Diagnosis

### *Differential diagnosis*

- Cauda equina syndrome
- Pachymeningitis hypertrophica
- Spinal cord tumor

### *History*

- Burning sensation in the sacral region
- Severe pain down the back of the legs
- Nonsciatic-type pain
- Burning at the medial knees
- Pain and tingling in the feet
- Mobility may be severely restricted

### *Exam*

- Paraspinal tenderness
- Positive straight leg raise
- Muscle atrophy
- Muscle spasm
- Decreased ankle reflexes
- Extremity weakness

### *Testing*

- MRI demonstrates adherent nerve roots located centrally in the thecal sac, adherence of the nerve roots to

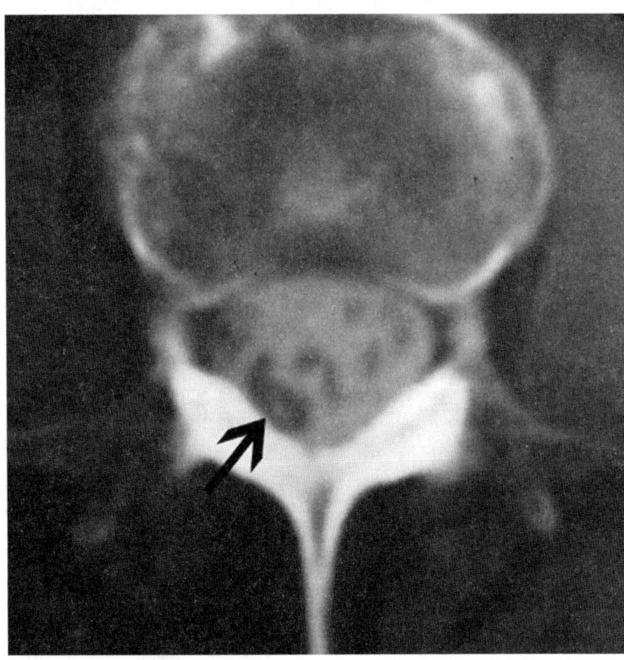

Axial lumbar computed tomography myelography demonstrating nerve root clumping (arrow) that is characteristic of arachnoiditis. (Adapted from Fast A, Goldsher D. *Navigating the Adult Spine: Bridging Clinical Practice and Neuroradiology.* New York: Demos Medical Publishing, 2007:140.)

the meninges, and a soft tissue mass that replaces the subarachnoid space.

- MRI with gadolinium does not demonstrate signal changes with arachnoiditis, allowing differentiation from neoplasm.
- Myelography demonstrates loculations of contrast dye, loss of nerve root sleeves, and partial or total obstruction of dye flow.

### *Pitfalls*

- None

## Red Flags

- Progressive cauda equina syndrome

## Treatment

### *Medical*

- Opioids for pain control
- Medications for neuropathic pain

### *Exercises*

- Exercise may be difficult due to pain
- Important to encourage as much physical activity as possible

### *Modalities*

- Heat, cold, ultrasound, and transcutaneous electrical nerve stimulation have been used for symptomatic relief of pain and muscle spasms.

### *Injection*

- Experimental use of intrathecal hyaluronidase
- Removal of residual oil-based contrast dye
- Epidural steroid injection for radicular symptoms
- Endoscopic lysis of adhesions

### *Surgical*

- Gentle handling of the neural elements during surgery can decrease the risk of development of adhesions.
- Spinal cord stimulation has demonstrated up to a 50% reduction in pain.
- Poor outcome with surgical intervention

### *Consults*

- Neurologic or orthopedic-spine surgery
- Physical medicine and rehabilitation
- Anesthesia

### *Complications of treatment*

- Cauda equine syndrome
- Arachnoiditis ossificans
- Partial or complete paralysis and numbness of the lower extremities
- Pain at rest
- Constant burning pain in the lower extremities
- Syringomyelia
- Rare progression to paraplegia or death

## Prognosis

- Constant severe pain with significant disability
- Bladder dysfunction may develop later in the course of the disease.
- Increased risk of depression, suicide, and substance abuse
- Life span may be decreased up to 12 years.

## Helpful Hints

- Poor response to analgesics

## Suggested Readings

Bourne IH. Lumbo-sacral adhesive arachnoiditis: a review. *J R Soc Med.* 1990;83(4):262–265.

Burton CV. Lumbosacral arachnoiditis. *Spine.* 1978;3(1):24–30.

Guyer DW, Wiltse LL, Eskay ML, Guyer BH. The long-range prognosis of arachnoiditis. *Spine.* 1989;14(12):1332–1341.

# Arteriovenous Malformation

## Description

An arteriovenous malformation (AVM) is an abnormal collection of high-pressure arteries and veins without intervening capillaries that may enlarge or rupture.

## Etiology/Types

- Glomerular types are the most common and are located superficially or within the spinal cord.
- Fistulous types are arteriovenous shunts most commonly found superficially on the spinal cord and are subcategorized into low- and high-shunt volume subtypes.

## Epidemiology

- Most common in patients over 30 years of age
- Male predominance

## Pathogenesis

- May be located throughout the spinal column
- Increased vascular pressure results in vessel enlargement resulting in spinal cord dysfunction.

## Risk Factors

- Hereditary hemorrhagic telangiectasia

## Clinical Features

- Exercise claudication
- Occasionally associated with cutaneous angioma
- Bruit may be heard with auscultation over the spine.
- Venous congestion is associated with chronic and progressive myelopathy.
- Neurologic deficits may also be associated with space-occupying AVMs.
- Acute or chronic neurologic deficits may be associated with intramedullary or subarachnoid hemorrhage.

## Natural History

- Progressive claudication, dysesthesias, and radicular pain
- Thrombosis of the vessels may result in symptom progression over several hours to weeks.
- Cervical AVM increases the risk of subarachnoid hemorrhage.

## Diagnosis

### *Differential diagnosis*

- Intramedullary spinal tumor

### *History*

- May be asymptomatic
- Variable neurological deficits ranging from radiculopathy to myelopathy

### *Exam*

- Variable neurological deficits ranging from radiculopathy to myelopathy

### *Testing*

- Spinal angiography is used for diagnosis and surgical planning.
- MRI may not always be able to identify an AVM.
- MRI can identify myelomalacia, edema, blood vessel thrombosis or thickening, and the presence of new bleeding

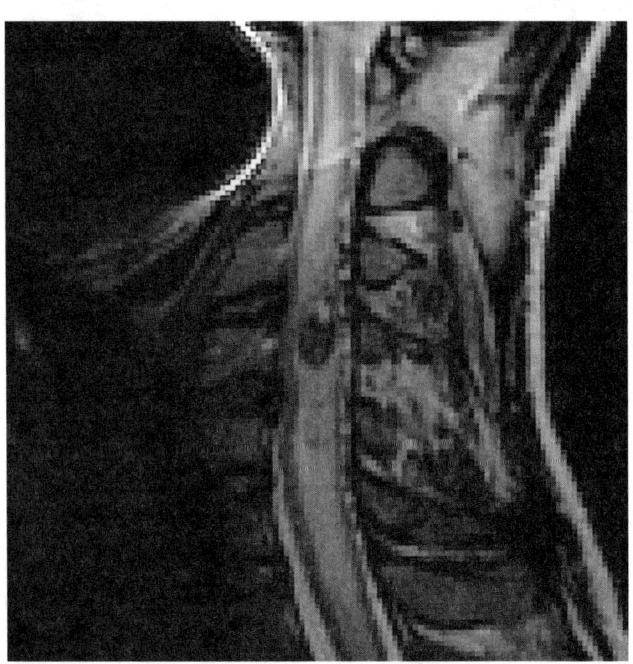

Sagittal cervical T2-weighted magnetic resonance image demonstrating an arteriovenous malformation within the spinal cord at the C4 level. (Adapted from Fast A, Goldsher D. *Navigating the Adult Spine: Bridging Clinical Practice and Neuroradiology.* New York: Demos Medical Publishing, 2007:130.)

- CSF analysis may be normal or demonstrate red blood cells and increased protein.
- Electrodiagnostic testing may demonstrate multiple scattered bilateral radiculopathies of the thoracic, lumbar, and sacral nerve roots.

### *Pitfalls*

- Chronic myelopathy related to venous congestion may present with nonspecific neurologic changes making diagnosis difficult.

## Red Flags

- Progressive neurologic deficits or myelopathy

## Treatment

### *Medical*

- None

### *Exercises*

- None

### *Modalities*

- None

### *Injection*

- None

### *Surgical*

- Asymptomatic AVMs should remain untreated.
- Surgical indications include progressive neurologic dysfunction and recurrent bleeding.
- Endovascular embolization
- Surgical resection with or without presurgical endovascular embolization

### *Consults*

- Neurologic or orthopedic-spine surgery

### *Complications of treatment*

- Endovascular embolization and surgery decreases the risk of bleeding but increases the risk of further neurologic deterioration.

## Prognosis

- There is no data on the progression of asymptomatic AVMs.

## Helpful Hints

- Progressive neurologic deficits or myelopathy should be evaluated and treated promptly.

## Suggested Readings

Bostroem A, Thron A, Hans FJ, Krings T. Spinal vascular malformations—typical and atypical findings. *Zentralbl Neurochir.* 2007;68(4):205–213.

*Zozulya YP, Slin'ko EI, Al-Qashqish II. Spinal arteriovenous malformations: new classification and surgical treatment. Neurosurg Focus. 2006;20(5):E7.*

# Atlantoaxial Instability

## Description

Atlantoaxial instability (AAI) is characterized by increased motion at the atlas (C1) and axis (C2) interface, resulting from a bony or ligamentous abnormality.

## Etiology/Types

Three patterns of instability are flexion–extension, distraction, and rotation.

## Epidemiology

- Unknown prevalence in the general population
- Only 16% of atlantoaxial injuries result in neurologic deficits due to a large central spinal canal at this level.
- 15% of individuals with Down syndrome have laxity of the transverse ligament.

## Pathogenesis

- Stability is mainly provided by the transverse ligament and the two modified zygapophyseal (facet) joints.
- The transverse ligament and the odontoid process are the most common structures involved in instability.
- The alar ligament and tectorial membrane resist vertical displacement.
- Symptoms develop when the odontoid process or posterior arch of the atlas impinges on the spinal cord.

## Risk Factors

- Cerebral palsy
- Down syndrome
- Dwarfism
- Grisel syndrome
- Klippel–Feil anomaly
- Larsen syndrome
- Neurofibromatosis
- Osteogenesis imperfecta
- Rheumatoid arthritis

## Clinical Features

- History of head trauma
- Occipital pain in patients with rheumatoid arthritis
- Myelopathy

## Natural History

- Asymptomatic patients with instability are not at higher risk of developing symptoms.

## Diagnosis

### *Differential diagnosis*

- Abnormal ossification or fracture of the odontoid
- Tumors

### *History*

- Neck and/or suboccipital pain
- Pain improved with supine positioning
- Pain worsened with cervical range of motion

### *Exam*

- Restricted neck range of motion
- Tenderness overlying the C1–C2 articulation
- Upper motor neuron findings with myelopathy

### *Testing*

- Open-mouth odontoid and lateral cervical spine X-rays
- Transverse ligament rupture is noted if the combined spread of the lateral masses of C1 on C2 exceeds 6.9 mm.
- Atlantodens interval (ADI) is the distance between the odontoid process and the posterior aspect of the anterior arch of the atlas measured on lateral X-rays.
  - Normally ≤3 mm in adults and ≤5 mm in children
  - Instability is present when there is an ADI difference of 3.5 mm or more on flexion/extension views.
- Posterior atlantodental interval (PADI) measures the space available in the central canal and is the distance from the posterior border of the dens to the anterior border of the posterior tubercle.
  - Correlates with the degree of neurological deficits
- CT and MRI can provide additional information on rotational AAI and spinal cord injury.

### *Pitfalls*

- Missed diagnosis

## Red Flags

- Myelopathy

## Treatment

### *Medical*

- Preparticipation sports physicals are recommended for patients at risk.
- The Special Olympics requires all children with Down syndrome to have neurologic and radiographic examinations to assess for AAI.

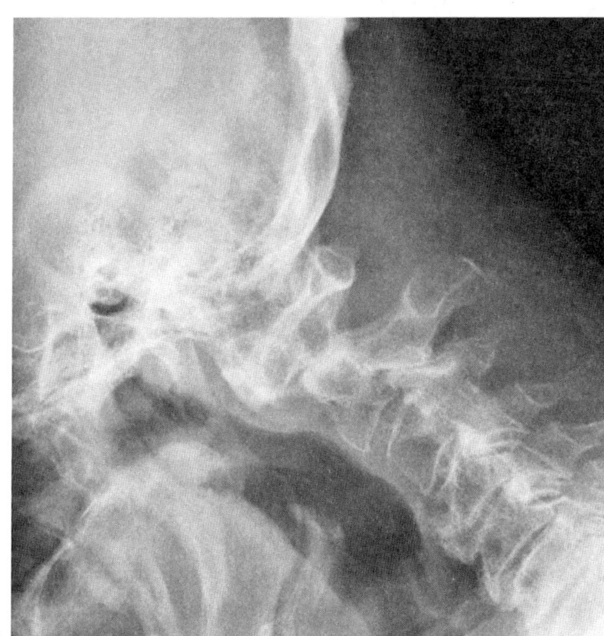

A

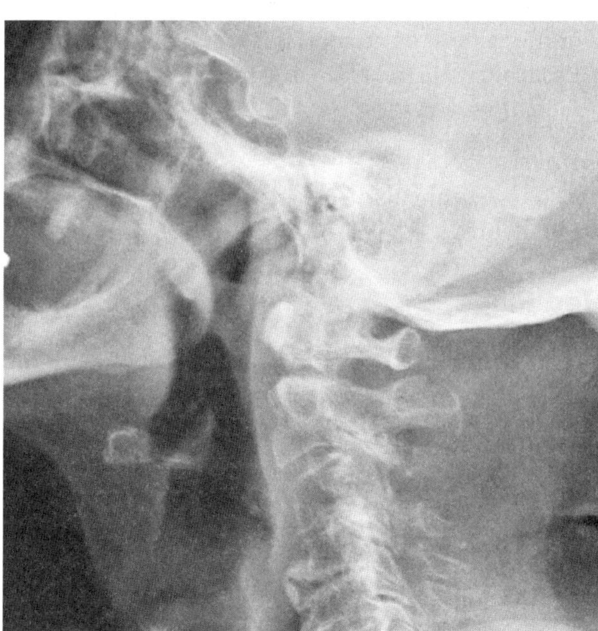

B

Lateral cervical flexion (A) and extension (B) plain radiographs demonstrating anterior subluxation of the odontoid process and the anterior arch of the atlas due to a fracture of the base of the odontoid process. (Courtesy of Keith Hentel, MD.)

### *Exercises*

- None

### *Modalities*

- None

### *Injection*

- None

### *Surgical*

- Posterior C1–C2 fusion is done with ligamentous injuries, as these ligaments have poor healing potential.
- Surgery is most effective in patients with severe pain and mild signs of myelopathy.
- Surgery is not recommended for patients without signs of myelopathy.
- The indication for surgery in rheumatoid arthritis patients are atlantoaxial subluxation of >8 mm with cord compression, PADI <14 mm, >3.5 mm subaxial subluxation, or progressive neurological deficit.
- Fusion is more extensive from the occiput to C2.

### *Consults*

- Neurologic or orthopedic-spine surgery
- Physical medicine and rehabilitation

### *Complications of treatment*

- Spinal cord injury

## Prognosis

- Symptomatic patients are at increased risk of developing further neurologic deficits, yet paralysis and death are rare.
- Good functional prognosis following fusion surgery
- Early identification of a progressive myelopathy improves the functional prognosis.

## Helpful Hints

- No treatment required unless there are signs of spinal cord injury or compression.

## Suggested Reading

Herman MJ, Pizzutillo PD. Cervical spine disorders in children. *Orthop Clin North Am.* 1999;30(3):457–466.

# Aviation-Associated Back and Neck Pain

## Description
Back and neck pain associated with aviation

## Etiology/Types
- Thought to be related to vibration, prolonged static positioning, and poor posture

## Epidemiology
- 92% of young healthy aviators report back pain.

## Pathogenesis
- Sustained high Gz (acceleration due to gravity) maneuvers for 40 minutes have been found to decrease body height 4.9 mm and increase the risk of injury due to decreased intervertebral segment elasticity.
- Vibration is thought to lead to intervertebral disc microtrauma, which may predispose the disc to further injury.
- Pilot seats in commercial aircraft were designed to withstand excessive forces during accidents, but do not reportedly meet basic ergonomic design criteria.
- Most coach seats do not meet basic ergonomic design criteria.

## Risk Factors
- Aircraft vibration during takeoff, landing, and turbulence
- Confined sitting position
- Helmet-mounted equipment
- Hoisting bags into overhead bins
- Physical deconditioning
- Prolonged static positioning
- Repeated exposure to accelerations exceeding 4.0 Gz
- Rushing through airports with heavy luggage

## Clinical Features
- Typically neck and lower back range of motion will be decreased due to pain or restriction related to axial spine degenerative changes or tissue inflexibility.
- Paraspinal muscle spasm

## Natural History
- Progressive pain and discomfort

## Diagnosis

### Differential diagnosis
- Ankylosing spondylitis
- Degenerative disc disease
- Osteoarthritis
- Osteoporosis
- Rheumatoid arthritis

### History
- Progressive pain and discomfort during flight

### Exam
- Normal motor, sensory, and reflex examinations
- Tenderness in the cervical or lumbar paraspinal muscles

### Testing
- Imaging is done if the pain persists for several weeks or if weakness or numbness is found on examination.
- Electrodiagnostic testing is used to assess for radiculopathy.

### Pitfalls
- Missing rheumatoid arthritis or ankylosing spondylitis

## Red Flags
- Severe weakness, numbness, or tingling
- Bowel or bladder dysfunction

## Treatment

### Medical
- NSAIDs and relative rest for 24 hours after an acute injury or exacerbation
- Prepositioning of the head and body prior to a high Gz maneuver
- Postural and equipment modifications
- Minimizing prolonged sitting during flight
- Use of a pillow or rolled blanket for lumbar or thigh support
- Luggage placed under the seat can be used as a footrest.
- Business and first class commercial airline travel allows greater room to adjust seating comfort.

### Exercises
- Routine neck and lower back stretching and strengthening program

### *Modalities*

- Heat, cold, ultrasound, and transcutaneous electrical nerve stimulation have been used for symptomatic relief of pain and muscle spasms.

### *Injection*

- Trigger point injections for symptoms of myofascial pain
- Epidural steroid injections for radicular symptoms

### *Surgical*

- Discectomy
- Fusion

### *Consults*

- Physical medicine and rehabilitation
- Neurologic or orthopedic-spine surgery
- General practitioner

### *Complications of treatment*

- Progressive debilitating pain

## Prognosis

- General aviation guidelines:
  - Pilots can return to flight duties once they are asymptomatic.
  - Pilots are disqualified from flying if their low back symptoms are recurrent or chronic, have required hospitalization, and require regular medication beyond NSAIDs.
- With nerve involvement or surgery, pilots will need to be asymptomatic for 6 weeks before they can be considered fit to return to flight status.
- Fusion surgery can result in pilots being grounded for 6 months.
- Pilots are permanently disqualified for multilevel discectomies.
- Passengers may have significant difficulty flying after multilevel discectomies due to seat ergonomics.

## Helpful Hints

- Early ergonomic modifications can safeguard against the development of a chronic pain condition.

## Suggested Reading

Mohler SR. Lower back pain is a common complaint, but precautionary practices help pilots cope. *Hum Factors Aviat Med Flight Safety Foundation.* 2000;47(3):1–6.

# Baastrup's Disease (Kissing Spines Disease)

## Description

Baastrup's disease is the development of a neoarthrosis between adjacent spinous processes.

## Etiology/Types

- Caused by breakdown of the interspinous ligament

## Epidemiology

- More common with advancing age
- Young athletes
- Prevalence on autopsy ranges from 6.2% to 22.1%
- Most common at the L4 to L5 level

## Pathogenesis

- The supraspinous and intraspinous ligaments are sprained with extreme forward flexion, which may result in the development of a spur.
- Repetitive extension may disrupt the healing process.
- An interspinous bursae may develop due to supraspinous ligament laxity and intraspinous ligament breakdown.
- The interspinous ligament degenerates with aging resulting in the formation of a cavity, which can precede the development of pain.

## Risk Factors

- Central spinal stenosis
- Degenerative disc disease
- Zygapophyseal (facet) joint osteoarthritis
- Gymnastics
- Hyperlordosis
- Paraspinal muscle atrophy
- Pars interarticularis defect

## Clinical Features

- Localized interspinous or spinous process pain with or without a referral pattern

## Natural History

- May be present for many years with progressive worsening over time
- The pain may be significant enough to limit activities of daily living.

## Diagnosis

### *Differential diagnosis*

- Central spinal canal stenosis
- Infection
- Lumbar spondylosis
- Muscle strain
- Paracentral disc herniation
- Spinous process fracture
- Spondylolisthesis
- Vertebral compression fracture

### *History*

- Localized interspinous or spinous process pain with or without a referral pattern

### *Exam*

- Difficult to assess proximity of spinous processes on manual palpation due to their overlapping nature
- Palpable tenderness of the supraspinous ligament with the patient in a side lying–fetal position
- Pain with extension > flexion

### *Testing*

- Lateral plain radiographs may demonstrate sclerotic changes or flattening of adjacent spinous processes
- MRI is useful to assess for interspinous edema or edema associated with early pars lesion; it can also rule out infection, tumor or a herniated disc.
- Bone scanning with single-photon emission computed tomography (SPECT) can detect increased osteoblastic activity that is associated with reactive sclerosis.

### *Pitfalls*

- Pars interarticularis fracture
- Spinous process fracture
- Vertebral compression fracture
- Lack of imaging findings

## Red Flags

- Infection

## Treatment

### *Medical*

- Bed rest in the semi-Fowler position (semiupright sitting position of 45 to 60 degrees with the knees either bent or straight)

### Exercises
- Gentle strengthening and stretching
- Flexion bias

### Modalities
- Heat, cold, ultrasound, and transcutaneous electrical nerve stimulation have been used for symptomatic relief of pain and muscle spasms.

### Injection
- Fluoroscopically guided diagnostic-interspinous injections have been used to confirm the diagnosis and for treatment.
  - Characteristic dye pattern is noted to be a cavity with a firm endpoint.
  - Injection may need to be repeated.

### Surgical
- Cavity resection
- Fusion

### Consults
- Physical medicine and rehabilitation
- Neurologic or orthopedic-spine surgery

### Complications of treatment
- Complications related to surgery

## Prognosis
- Unknown

## Helpful Hints
- A clinical diagnosis, without findings on imaging may also be treated effectively with a corticosteroid/ anesthetic infiltration.

## Suggested Readings
Haig AJ, Harris A, Quint DJ. Baastrup's disease correlating with diffuse lumbar paraspinal atrophy: a case report. *Arch Phys Med Rehabil.* 2001;82(2):250–252.

Mitra R, Ghazi U, Kirpalani D, Cheng I. Interspinous ligament steroid injections for the management of Baastrup's disease: a case report. *Arch Phys Med Rehabil.* 2007;88(10):1353–1356.

# Back Pain Associated with Dance

## Description

Back pain or injury that develops during dance training or performance

## Etiology/Types

- Related to age and skill

## Epidemiology

- Male predominance
- Spondylolysis is four times as common in dancers as compared to the general population.
- Increased incidence of spondylolysis with vigorous performance or rehearsals

## Pathogenesis

- Repetitive microtrauma
- Injuries related to hyperlordosis occur with turning, jumping, or lifting.
- Male dancers develop upper back pain from strains due to lifting.

## Risk Factors

- Growth spurt resulting in decreased flexibility and musculotendinous tightening
- Hip joint abnormalities
- Hyperlordosis
- Improper footwear
- Leg-length discrepancies
- Musculotendinous imbalance
- Patellar misalignment
- Pes planus
- Training errors or significant changes in dance style, intensity, and frequency

## Clinical Features

- Hamstring tightness
- Pain from a pars interarticularis fracture is worsened with extension, especially in the arabesque position.
- Localized paraspinal muscle spasm
- Step off related to a spondylolisthesis

## Natural History

- Progressive pain

## Diagnosis

### *Differential diagnosis*

- Chondroplasia
- Discogenic back pain
- Infection
- Inflammatory spondyloarthropathies
- Neoplasm
- Sacroiliac joint pain
- Spondylolisthesis
- Spondylolysis
- Spondylosis

### *History*

- Progressive pain during training or performance

### *Exam*

- Pain from a pars interarticularis fracture is worsened with extension
- Localized paraspinal muscle spasm
- Hamstring tightness
- Stepoff related to a spondylolisthesis

### *Testing*

- X-rays should include oblique views to assess for pars interarticularis fractures.
- SPECT scan is indicated when there is a high suspicion of a pars interarticularis fracture with normal plain radiographs.
- CT scan may also be used to assess zygapophyseal (facet) joint irregularity.
- MRI is used to assess for stress fractures.

### *Pitfalls*

- Convincing dancers to decrease their dance intensity, duration, and frequency

## Red Flags

- Undiagnosed fracture
- Radicular symptoms
- Unrelenting pain

## Treatment

### *Medical*

- Assessment of a dancer's technique and dance style to manage and prevent reinjury
- Dancers with disabling pain or progressive neurologic decline should be managed as the general population.
- Conservative treatment with grades 1 and 2 and asymptomatic grade 3 spondylolisthesis

### Exercises

- Upper body and core abdominal muscle strengthening to decrease hyperlordosis and improve lifting technique
- Antilordotic brace that is worn full time for 4 to 6 months but removed during training in dancers with a tight lordosis
- Spondylolysis of less than 6 months duration is immobilized with an antilordotic brace.
- Pilates

### Modalities

- Muscle strains that occur during a performance may be treated with an ice massage or cold spray for symptomatic relief.
- Heat, ultrasound, and transcutaneous electrical nerve stimulation have been used for symptomatic relief of pain and muscle spasms.

### Injection

- Trigger point injections for symptoms of myofascial pain
- Epidural steroid injections for radicular symptoms

### Surgical

- Discectomy
- If pain from a pars fracture continues to be unresponsive to conservative treatments, fusion may be considered.
- Surgical debridement of a pars interarticularis nonunion
- Fusion is considered in symptomatic grade 3 and grade 4 spondylolistheses.

### Consults

- Physical medicine and rehabilitation
- Neurologic or orthopedic-spine surgery

### Complications of treatment

- Dancers' inability to return to their preinjury level of dance
- Complications related to surgery

## Prognosis

- Following discectomy, dancers may not be able to perform for up to one year.
- Return to professional dance will depend on the degree of recovery.
- Spondylolysis with grade 1 spondylolisthesis will remain stable and dancers can continue to dance safely although pain may be problematic.

## Helpful Hints

- Prevention is important.
- Lordotic posturing should be monitored by dance instructors.
- Emphasis on core abdominal strengthening

## Suggested Readings

Hansen PA, Reed K. Common musculoskeletal problems in the performing artist. *Phys Med Rehabil Clin N Am.* 2006;17(4):789–801.

Micheli LJ. Back injuries in dancers. *Clin Sports Med.* 1983;2(3):473–484.

# Back Pain Associated with Golf

## Description

Back pain that develops during participation in golf

## Etiology/Types

- The golf swing generates a large rotational force that is controlled by the annulus fibrosis, zygapophyseal (facet) joints, musculotendinous, and fascial thoracolumbar stabilizers.

## Epidemiology

- Low back pain represents 26% to 52% of all golf-related injuries.
- 30% of touring professional golfers play with low back pain

## Pathogenesis

- A golf swing requires lateral bending with axial compression and torsion, which is the most common cause of disc herniation.
  - The annulus fibrosis and zygapophyseal (facet) joints limit rotation.
  - Protective reflexive muscle stabilization can diminish with repetitive loading, resulting in creep and progressive laxity.
  - Laxity and decreased coordination of the thoracolumbar fascial stabilizers increases risk of injury.
- In professional golfers, axial compression during a golf swing at the L3–L4 segment can be up to eight times body weight (7,584 ± 2,422 N).
  - Disc prolapse in cadaveric studies can occur with only 5,448 N of axial compression.
- Four basic components of the golf swing are the backswing, forward swing, acceleration with ball strike, and follow-through.
- The modern golf swing, which generates greater force and distance, increases the hip–shoulder separation angle with a large shoulder turn and a restricted hip turn.
- The classic golf swing reduces the hip–shoulder separation angle and the torque on the axial spine by raising the heel to increase the hip turn or shortening the backswing alone or in combination.

## Risk Factors

- Carrying a golf bag during play
- Constant practice sessions
- Decreased lead hip internal rotation
- Osteoporotic vertebral body compression fractures
- Poor biomechanics resulting in greater torque and shear forces in amateurs
- Trunk muscle imbalance

## Clinical Features

- Axial low back pain
- Pain with extension or rotation
- Pain during a golf swing

## Natural History

- Progressive pain

## Diagnosis

### *Differential diagnosis*

- Central spinal stenosis
- Degenerative disc disease
- Fracture
- Herniated nucleus pulposus
- Neoplasm or metastasis
- Radiculopathy

### *History*

- Axial low back pain with or without radiation

### *Exam*

- Pain with extension or rotation
- Pain during a golf swing
- Paraspinal muscle spasm
- Poor truncal strength
- Decreased quadriceps or hamstring flexibility
- Decreased hip range of motion

### *Testing*

- X-rays may be used to assess for degenerative changes or fracture, but can be nonspecific.
- CT may be helpful in further delineating the bony anatomy or fracture.
- MRI can be used to assess the intervertebral discs, nerve roots. and ligaments.
- Electrodiagnostic testing can be used to assess for radiculopathy.

### *Pitfalls*

- Missed fracture

## Red Flags

- Radiculopathy

- Fracture
- Bowel or bladder dysfunction

## Treatment

### Medical

- Swing modifications
- Gradual return with swinging short irons, practicing on the driving range, and trialing a 9-hole game prior to full 18 holes
- Defer shots from deep rough, sand, or angled lies
- During recovery, players should ride a golf cart or walk with a pull cart.

### Exercises

- General strengthening and stretching with emphasis on core abdominal strengthening
- Dynamic stabilization exercises targeting the transverse abdominus and multifidi muscles
- Flexibility training in the older population

### Modalities

- Heat, cold, ultrasound, and transcutaneous electrical nerve stimulation have been used for symptomatic relief of pain and muscle spasms.

### Injection

- Trigger point injections for symptoms of myofascial pain
- Epidural steroid injection for radicular symptoms
- Medial branch blocks/radiofrequency neurotomy for zygapophyseal (facet) joint–mediated pain

### Surgical

- Fusion

### Consults

- Physical medicine and rehabilitation
- Neurologic or orthopedic-spine surgery

### Complications of treatment

- Adjacent level disease following lumbar fusion may be accelerated with golfing activities.

## Prognosis

- Following a laminectomy, a player can begin swinging a club at 6 to 12 weeks.
- Lumbar fusion patients are restricted from swinging a club for at least 6 to 12 months postoperatively.

## Helpful Hints

- Golf is not a benign sport.

## Suggested Readings

Gluck GS, Bendo JA, Spivak JM. The lumbar spine and low back pain in golf: a literature review of swing biomechanics and injury prevention. *Spine J.* 2007.

Parziale JR, Mallon WJ. Golf injuries and rehabilitation. *Phys Med Rehabil Clin N Am.* 2006;17(3):589–607.

# Back Pain Associated with Heavy Loads

## Description

Back pain related to lifting or maneuvering heavy loads

## Etiology/Types

- Repetitive lifting changes muscle recruitment patterns resulting in poor spinal loading patterns, which increases the risk of injury.

## Epidemiology

- 33% of all work-related back pain events are caused by lifting or bending.

## Pathogenesis

- Squat lift, with the knees bent and back straight, is considered safer than the stoop lift, with the knees straight and back bent.
  - Minimal research supports the squat lift over the stoop lift.
- Most workers prefer the stoop lift as the squat lift results in more rapid fatigue.
  - Greater extensor muscle activity results in greater fatigue due to repetitive or sustained loading.
- Increased muscle activity and/or an increased intra-abdominal pressure increases spinal stability.
- Momentary loss of spinal stability can lead to unexpected displacement in the spine, resulting in injury.

## Risk Factors

- Awkward posture
- Cognitive, emotional, and psychosocial factors
- Fatigue
- High-stress work environment
- Increased trunk velocity
- Inadequate lifting strength of an individual compared to the occupational lifting demands
- Lifting with twisting or lateral bending
- Low job satisfaction
- Poor social support
- Very heavy loads

## Clinical Features

- Patients primarily complain of axial low back pain with or without radiation into the lower extremities.
- Hypertrophy of the paraspinal extensor group indicates increased load on these muscles.
- Associated with pain complaints in other regions of the body

## Natural History

- Progressive axial low back pain

## Diagnosis

### *Differential diagnosis*

- Central spinal stenosis
- Degenerative disc disease
- Fracture
- Herniated nucleus pulposus
- Neoplasm or metastasis
- Radiculopathy

### *History*

- Axial low back pain
- Muscle spasm

### *Exam*

- Decreased lumbar flexion and extension due to pain
- Body asymmetry
- Tenderness to palpation of the paraspinal muscles
- Paraspinal hypertrophy

### *Testing*

- Not generally required in nonspecific low back pain, although important if pain has not improved within 4 to 6 weeks.
- Usefulness of MRI in nonspecific low back pain is questionable, as degenerative findings are common in asymptomatic subjects.
- Electrodiagnostic study to assess for a radiculopathy

### *Pitfalls*

- Increasing time off from work

## Red Flags

- Bowel or bladder dysfunction
- Fracture
- Radiculopathy

## Treatment

### *Medical*

- Ergonomic assessment of the work-station or workplace
- Short-term NSAIDs

### *Exercises*

- Training programs can reduce the incidence of back pain in the workplace.

- Work hardening may be indicated to strengthen weak muscles.
- Proper lifting instruction
- Instructions in safe lifting techniques should include a plan for the lift, keeping the load close to the body, avoiding twisting, and bending at the knees.

### *Modalities*
- Heat, cold, ultrasound, and transcutaneous electrical nerve stimulation have been used for symptomatic relief of pain and muscle spasms.

### *Injection*
- Trigger point injections for symptoms of myofascial pain
- Epidural injections for symptoms related to radiculitis or stenosis

### *Surgical*
- None

### *Consults*
- Physical medicine and rehabilitation

### *Complications of treatment*
- Progressive work disability

## Prognosis
- The prognosis can be good if the causes are related to ergonomic factors or lack of body mechanics or body awareness with lifting.
- Poor prognosis if psychosocial or social factors play a significant role and are not addressed.

## Helpful Hints
- Address workplace ergonomics and possible additional psychosocial stressors that may be contributing factors.

## Suggested Readings
Arjmand N, Shirazi-Adl A. Biomechanics of changes in lumbar posture in static lifting. *Spine.* 2005;30(23):2637–2648.

Schenk P, et al. Symptomatology of recurrent low back pain in nursing and administrative professions. *Eur Spine J.* 2007.

# Back Pain Associated with Occupation

## Description

Back pain associated with tasks in the workplace

## Etiology/Types

- Generally unknown

## Epidemiology

- Most common cause of disability in adults aged 45 years or younger
- Patients covered by worker's compensation plans tend to have greater health care utilization and a longer duration of recovery compared to other forms of insurance.

## Pathogenesis

- Low back strain
- Radiculopathy
- Zygapophyseal (facet) joint pain

## Risk Factors

- Bending
- Cognitive, emotional, and psychosocial factors
- High-stress work environment
- Inadequate lifting strength of an individual compared to the occupational lifting demands
- Low job satisfaction
- Manual lifting
- Poor social support
- Smoking
- Twisting
- Very heavy loads
- Whole body vibration

## Clinical Features

- Patients primarily complain of axial low back pain with or without radiation into the lower extremities.
- Hypertrophy of the paraspinal extensor group indicates increased load on these muscles.

## Natural History

- Progressive axial low back pain

## Diagnosis

### *Differential diagnosis*

- Central spinal stenosis
- Degenerative disc disease
- Fracture
- Herniated nucleus pulposus
- Neoplasm or metastasis
- Radiculopathy

### *History*

- Difficult to ascertain work relatedness, the recurrence of a previous injury, or the onset of a systemic illness
- Review previous visits to the emergency room or hospital stays

### *Exam*

- Decreased lumbar flexion and extension due to pain
- Paraspinal hypertrophy
- Tenderness to palpation of the paraspinal muscles
- Body asymmetry
- Waddell's nonorganic signs (distraction. overreaction, regionalization, simulation, and tenderness)

### *Testing*

- Not generally required in nonspecific low back pain, although important if pain has not improved within 4 to 6 weeks.
- The usefulness of MRI in nonspecific low back pain is questionable as degenerative findings are common in asymptomatic subjects.

### *Pitfalls*

- An inadequate history and physical examination can lead to poor treatment outcomes and recurrent injury.
- Pending or ongoing litigation acts as an incentive to minimize recovery, continue diagnostic testing, and overvalue surgical intervention.

## Red Flags

- Associated febrile illness
- Cauda equina syndrome
- Fracture
- Numbness or tingling
- Weakness

## Treatment

### *Medical*

- Advice to remain active
- NSAIDs

- Muscle relaxants
- Analgesics
- Workstation assessment
- Acupuncture has been described as being helpful.

### Exercises

- Initial passive treatments should progress to active strengthening and stretching with a major emphasis on developing a home exercise program.

### Modalities

- Heat, cold, ultrasound, and transcutaneous electrical nerve stimulation have been used for symptomatic relief of pain and muscle spasms.

### Injection

- Trigger point injections for symptoms of myofascial pain
- Epidural steroid injection for radicular symptoms

### Surgical

- None acutely unless there is a surgical lesion

### Consults

- Referral to a multidisciplinary rehabilitation program, if there is difficulty returning to work after 4 to 12 weeks
- Physical medicine and rehabilitation
- Neurologic or orthopedic-spine surgery for clear surgical pathology

### Complications of treatment

- Inability to return to preinjury occupation

## Prognosis

- 85% of the total medical costs result from only 10% of patients with back pain of >3 months duration.
- Most patients with low back pain will recover within 4 to 6 weeks.
- 85% of patients will have symptom recurrence over their lifetime.
- A worker with a poor evaluation from an immediate supervisor within 6 months is most predictive of poor return to work status.

## Helpful Hints

- Complete pain relief should not be a limiting factor for return to work.

## Suggested Readings

Bigos SJ, Battie MC, Spengler DM, et al. A longitudinal, prospective study of industrial back injury reporting. *Clin Orthop Relat Res.* 1992;(279):21–34.

Nadler S, Stitik T. Occupational low back pain: history and physical examination. *Occup Med.* 1998;13(1):61–81.

# Back Pain Associated with Pregnancy

## Description

Back pain that is related to the unique changes associated with pregnancy

## Etiology/Types

- Ligamentous laxity due to the hormone relaxin
- Sacroiliac joint dysfunction
- Lumbar disc herniation
- Degenerative spondylolisthesis

## Epidemiology

- Estimates vary widely
- Incidence rate of low back pain in pregnancy can approach 50%.
- 30% to 45% of women in the postpartum period report low back pain.

## Pathogenesis

- Gravid uterus causes compensatory lumbar lordosis resulting in mechanical strain on the lower back and increased pelvic rotation.
- Relaxin is secreted by the corpus luteum resulting in ligamentous laxity and relaxation of the pelvic and sacroiliac joints.
- Prolonged supine positioning leads to obstruction of the vena cava, allowing venous congestion and hypoxemia, resulting in the development of lumbar pain.
- Lumbar disc herniation is the proximal source of pain in 1 in 10,000 cases of pregnancy-associated back pain.
- Pregnancy may also accelerate the development of a degenerative spondylolisthesis.

## Risk Factors

- Increasing maternal age
- Number of previous births
- Previous history of back pain with pregnancy

## Clinical Features

- Most common during the fifth to seventh month of pregnancy
- 46% describe radiation in the lower extremities
- Pain worsened with standing, sitting, forward flexion, lifting, and walking.

## Natural History

- Increasing pain with pregnancy that generally improves postpartum

## Diagnosis

### Differential diagnosis

- Discogenic pain
- Hip joint pathology
- Lumbar disc herniation
- Mechanical strain
- Pelvic ligamentous laxity
- Sacroiliac joint pain
- Spondylolisthesis

### History

- Lumbar of pelvic/sacroiliac pain with possible posterior thigh or inguinal radiation
- Improved with sitting, recumbency, or the use of a supportive pillow

### Exam

- Positive sacroiliac compression test
- Pain with bilateral compression over the iliac crests
- Positive Patrick's test
- Paraspinal muscle spasm
- Step-off deformity with spondylolisthesis

### Testing

- Noncontrast MRI may be performed with no recognized harm to the developing fetus; long-term consequences are unknown.

### Pitfalls

- Diagnosis is primarily based on clinical examination due to limitations of additional testing.

## Red Flags

- Bowel and bladder dysfunction
- Cauda equina syndrome
- Infection
- Weakness, numbness, or tingling

## Treatment

### Medical

- Activity and postural modifications
- Abdominal binders that help support the uterus
- Sacroiliac joint belt to stabilize the sacroiliac joint
- Oral pain medication should be coordinated with the obstetrician.
- Antiprostaglandins are contraindicated during pregnancy as they may cause a premature closure of the ductus arteriosus.

- Acetaminophen is often the pain reliever of choice.

### *Exercises*

- Exercise program focused on muscle imbalance and alignment of the pelvic girdle
- Pelvic tilts
- Aquatic exercise
- Sacroiliac joint mobilization

### *Modalities*

- Heat, transcutaneous electrical nerve stimulation, ultrasound are contraindicated.

### *Injection*

- Could consider an intralaminar epidural steroid without fluoroscopic guidance by an experienced practitioner

### *Surgical*

- Discectomy
- Laminectomy

### *Consults*

- Physical medicine and rehabilitation
- Neurologic or orthopedic-spine surgery for cauda equina or progressive neurologic deterioration

### *Complications of treatment*

- Postpartum weakness, numbness, or tingling

## Prognosis

- Very good prognosis for improvement within the first weeks after delivery
- Biopsychosocial factors may play a role in determining prognosis.

## Helpful Hints

- Regular exercise before pregnancy can reduce the risk of back pain.

## Suggested Readings

Bastiaanssen JM, de Bie RA, Bastiaenen CH, Essed GG, van den Brandt PA. A historical perspective on pregnancy-related low back and/or pelvic girdle pain. *Eur J Obstet Gynecol Reprod Biol.* 2005;120(1):3–14.

Borg-Stein J, Dugan S, Gruber J. Musculoskeletal aspects of pregnancy. *Am J Phys Med Rehabil.* 2005;84:180–192.

Fast A, Shapiro D, Ducommun EJ, Friedmann LW, Bouklas T, Floman Y. Low-back pain in pregnancy. *Spine.* 1987;12(4):368–371.

# Back Pain Associated with Sitting

## Description

Back pain associated with prolonged sitting or sitting on improper surfaces

## Etiology/Types

- Multifactorial

## Epidemiology

- 75% of workers in industrialized countries are involved in sedentary jobs that require prolonged sitting.

## Pathogenesis

- No evidence that sitting up "straight" or having "good posture" with a lumbar support is beneficial, although it is generally advised.
- Lower incidence of lumbar disc degeneration in populations that sit or squat with a compensatory flattening of the lumbar lordosis.
- Inactivity related with prolonged sitting is thought to decrease fluid flow across the endplates resulting in the accumulation of intradiscal metabolic byproducts causing accelerated disc degeneration.
- Prolonged sitting leads to static loading of soft tissues.
- Loss of the protective stabilizing reflexes of the multifidi with stretching of the viscoelastic structures
- Reclined seating allows some body weight to be transferred to the back rest and reinforces the lumbar lordosis.
- Intradiscal pressures are 35% higher, if sitting with no lumbar support as compared with standing.
- The work task has a great influence on muscle activity and lumbar disc pressure.

## Risk Factors

- Awkward posture
- Decreased physical conditioning
- Driving may be a risk factor
- Tall stature
- Obesity
- Pregnancy
- Prolonged sitting
- Psychological and physiological stress
- Smoking
- Whole body vibration

## Clinical Features

- Axial low back pain that is worsened with sitting

## Natural History

- Progressive axial low back pain

## Diagnosis

### *Differential diagnosis*

- Central spinal stenosis
- Degenerative disc disease
- Fracture
- Herniated nucleus pulposus
- Neoplasm or metastasis

### *History*

- Low back pain with sitting
- Low back pain that is better in the morning, worsens as the day progresses or with prolonged sitting

### *Exam*

- Rounded shoulders and a head forward posture with sitting
- Significant hamstring tightness is common
- Ely's test often uncovers quadriceps tightness
- Pain-limited lumbar flexion and extension
- Poor core stabilization demonstrated by uncoordinated hip extension while prone; normally there should be activity first at the erector spinae, followed by the gluteus medius, then the muscles of the hamstring complex.

### *Testing*

- Not generally required in nonspecific low back pain although important if pain has not improved within 4 to 6 weeks.
- The usefulness of MRI in nonspecific low back pain is questionable as degenerative findings are common in asymptomatic subjects

### *Pitfalls*

- Not addressing the seated work environment during the initial clinical visit

## Red Flags

- Bowel or bladder dysfunction
- Fracture
- Infection
- Radiculopathy

## Treatment

### *Medical*

- Sitting posture factors include the design of the chair, routine sitting habits, seat height and inclination, the position of the back rest, other supports as well as the work task.
- Chair design should include lumbar support and allow the occupant to easily adjust the seating surface.
- Use of arm rests and lumbar support reduce the pressure on the lumbar spine.
- Whole body vibration can be reduced using vibration isolation seats.
- Poor driver visibility and poor positioning of the controls requiring increased twisting and stretching should be addressed.
- Acupuncture has been described to be helpful.

### *Exercises*

- General strengthening and stretching with emphasis on core abdominal strengthening to maintain good strength and endurance as well as coordination

### *Modalities*

- Heat, cold, ultrasound, and transcutaneous electrical nerve stimulation have been used for symptomatic relief of pain and muscle spasms.

### *Injection*

- Trigger point injections for symptoms of myofascial pain

### *Surgical*

- None

### *Consults*

- Physical medicine and rehabilitation
- Ergonomist

### *Complications of treatment*

- Continued progressive axial low back pain

## Prognosis

- The prognosis is good if the underlying factors are identified.

## Helpful Hints

- Prevention is important.

## Suggested Readings

Lis AM, Black KM, Korn H, Nordin M. Association between sitting and occupational LBP. *Eur Spine J.* 2007;16(2):283–298.

Pope MH, Goh KL, Magnusson ML. Spine ergonomics. *Annu Rev Biomed Eng.* 2002;4:49–68.

# Back Pain Associated with Soccer

## Description

Back pain that occurs with participation in the sport of soccer

## Etiology/Types

- Cyclic loading with repetitive activities
- Muscle sprain or strains are the most common.
- Spondylosis
- Spondylolisthesis
- Spondylolysis
- Sacroiliac joint dysfunction

## Epidemiology

- Soccer is the fastest growing sport in the United States and the most popular sport in the world.
- Low back pain is the third most common soccer injury after knee and ankle injuries, respectively.

## Pathogenesis

- Players often note that their pain begins after a high-velocity kick.
- Sprains result from eccentric overload of the paraspinal muscles.
- Hip extension strength is often weaker following an episode of low back pain, increasing the risk of further injury.

## Risk Factors

- Decreased abdominal core strengthening
- Hamstring strength imbalance (hip extensor strength)
- Leg-length discrepancy
- Prior back strain
- Sacroiliac joint rotation

## Clinical Features

- Muscle strain or sprain results in localized muscle pain or spasm.
- Spondylosis, spondylolisthesis, or spondylolysis can refer pain to the buttocks or posterior thigh with rare radiation below the knee.

## Natural History

- Axial low back pain may resolve or progressively worsen

## Diagnosis

### *Differential diagnosis*

- Central spinal stenosis
- Degenerative disc disease
- Fracture
- Herniated nucleus pulposus
- Lumbar paraspinal sprain or strain
- Neoplasm or metastasis
- Radiculopathy

### *History*

- Pain worsened with running or kicking

### *Exam*

- Hip extensor strength imbalance
- Stepoff deformity associated with spondylolisthesis

### *Testing*

- Anteroposterior (AP) and lateral X-rays allow for assessment of vertebral body listhesis or dislocation.
- Oblique X-rays can assess osteoarthritic changes in the zygapophyseal (facet) joints or a defect of the pars interarticularis.
- MRI is useful to look at soft tissue elements of the spine including the ligaments and intervertebral discs.
- SPECT is used to detect a clinically suspected spondylolysis that has not been found on X-rays.
- Electrodiagnostic studies are useful in assessing for a potential radiculopathy.

### *Pitfalls*

- Diagnostic difficulty

## Red Flags

- Radiculopathy
- Fracture
- Bowel or bladder dysfunction

## Treatment

### *Medical*

- Heel lift for a leg-length discrepancy
- Sacroiliac joint mobilization
- Thoracolumbar bracing, commonly the use of a Boston brace, may be used for pain control in spondylolysis/spondylolisthesis.
- The bracing would have to be worn for 23 hours of the day.
- Acupuncture has been described to be helpful with associated muscle spasm.

### *Exercises*

- Core abdominal stabilization exercises to allow the player to stabilize the lumbopelvic region

- Hamstring strengthening with a focus on developing symmetric strength
- Training focused on developing endurance and power

### *Modalities*

- Heat, cold, ultrasound, and transcutaneous electrical nerve stimulation have been used for symptomatic relief of pain and muscle spasms.

### *Injection*

- Trigger point injections for symptoms of myofascial pain
- Epidural steroid injection for radicular symptoms

### *Surgical*

- Laminectomy for radiculopathy
- Repair of the pars interarticularis for spondylolysis

### *Consults*

- Physical medicine and rehabilitation
- Neurologic or orthopedic-spine surgery

### *Complications of treatment*

- Progression of the a stress fracture to a full pars interarticularis fracture

## Prognosis

- Spondylolysis requires the discontinuation of participation for 3 months.
- Discontinuation of the sport can be more effective than bracing.
- 78% to 92% of young participants with spondylolysis are able to return to full activities, but only 18% to 37% demonstrated evidence of bony healing.

## Helpful Hints

- The most common injury is a muscle strain or sprain.
- Spondylolysis is common in the soccer player due to the repetitive lumbar extension.
- Important to assess hamstring flexibility and strength

## Suggested Readings

El Rassi G, Takemitsu M, Woratanarat P, Shah SA. Lumbar spondylolysis in pediatric and adolescent soccer players. *Am J Sports Med.* 2005;33(11):1688–1693.

Manning MR, Levy RS. Soccer. *Phys Med Rehabil Clin N Am.* 2006;17(3):677–695.

# Back Pain Associated with Tennis

## Description

Back pain that occurs with participation in the sport of tennis

## Etiology/Types

- Continuous microtrauma from repetitive loading and rotation with hyperextension

## Epidemiology

- 38% of 148 professional tennis players missed a tournament due to back pain.
- Unknown if tennis players have a higher risk of back pain compared to the general population.

## Pathogenesis

- The serve causes the greatest stress on the lumbar spine.
- Traditional forehand groundstroke results in 90 degrees of axial spine rotation.
- The open-stanced forearm swing involves more rotational acceleration as there is less trunk rotation.
- The one-handed backhand requires less trunk rotation as the hitting shoulder is already facing the net.
- Grass courts and increased ball speed increase axial hyperextension.
- Zygapophyseal (facet) joint arthropathy on imaging was found in 70% of asymptomatic elite young tennis players, mean age 17 years, compared to 8% to 21% found in an asymptomatic general population with a mean age of 35 to 43 years.
- Pars interarticularis stress injuries are the second most common type of injuries in tennis due to excessive hyperextension during the serve.
- Disc degeneration in young elite tennis players is similar to nonelite athletes
- Spondylolisthesis occurs in 6% of asymptomatic elite young players.
- Asymmetrical loading occurs due to the forces generated by the dominant hitting shoulder on the nondominant side of the trunk, resulting in increased strength in the dominant forearm and increased external rotation with decreased internal rotation of the dominant shoulder.
- Smooth rotation with flexion–extension occurs through alternating and coordinated concentric–eccentric muscle action.

## Risk Factors

- Hamstring injury or inflexibility
- Lumbar inflexibility
- Muscle fatigue
- Repetitive muscle contraction
- Shoulder injury

## Clinical Features

- Lumbar strain results from a change in the intensity, duration, or technique during play.
- Sudden onset of symptoms; sometimes the onset of pain may follow a change in the normal routine after only a short period of time.

## Natural History

- Axial low back pain may resolve or progressively worsen.

## Diagnosis

### *Differential diagnosis*

- Degenerative disc disease
- Herniated nucleus pulposus
- Pars interarticularis stress reaction
- Radiculopathy
- Spondylolisthesis
- Spondylolysis
- Spondylosis

### *History*

- Lumbar strain or spondylosis may present as unilateral or bilateral lower back pain with or without a referral pattern.

### *Exam*

- Lumbar shift away from the painful side
- Concave spinal curvature toward the side of pain
- Symmetry of the posterior superior iliac spines should be documented.
- Lumbar flexion may be pain limited
- Pain free lumbar extension if the zygapophyseal (facet) joints are not affected
- Shoulder range of motion should be assessed.

### *Testing*

- Imaging is considered in patients with chronic back pain or signs of nerve root involvement.
- Oblique X-rays are used to assess the zygapophyseal (facet) joints.

- MRI is useful in assessing acute or chronic pars interarticularis injuries and to determine healing potential.
- Electrodiagnostic studies should be completed on players with neurologic deficits.

### Pitfalls

- Diagnostic difficulty

## Red Flags

- Radiculopathy
- Fracture
- Bowel or bladder dysfunction

## Treatment

### Medical

- Acute pars interarticularis stress responses can be limited with refraining from play.
- Injuries of the pars interarticularis respond better to treatment if recognized early.
- NSAIDs
- Analgesics
- Bracing for pars interarticularis fractures
- Acupuncture has been described as helpful for associated muscle spasm.

### Exercises

- General strengthening and stretching with emphasis on core abdominal strengthening
- Dynamic stabilization exercises with emphasis on strengthening of the muscles in the shoulder and lower extremities as well as the core abdominal muscles

### Modalities

- Heat, cold, ultrasound, and transcutaneous electrical nerve stimulation have been used for symptomatic relief of pain and muscle spasms.

### Injection

- Trigger point injections
- Epidural steroid injection for radicular symptoms

### Surgical

- Laminectomy for radiculopathy
- Repair of the pars interarticularis for spondylolysis

### Consults

- Physical medicine and rehabilitation
- Neurologic or orthopedic-spine surgery, if there has been no improvement with conservative treatment.

### Complications of treatment

- Progression of a pars interarticularis stress response to a full fracture

## Prognosis

- A player may return to play within several days after an uncomplicated acute lumbar strain.

## Helpful Hints

- Acute pars interarticularis stress responses can be limited with refraining from play.
- Emphasis on dynamic stabilization exercises for strengthening the shoulder stabilizer muscles, lower extremities, and the core abdominal muscles that connect these two areas.

## Suggested Reading

Perkins RH, Davis D. Musculoskeletal injuries in tennis. *Phys Med Rehabil Clin N Am.* 2006;17(3):609–631.

# Back Pain in Mature Athletes

## Description

Back pain that occurs in mature populations that engage in sports

## Etiology/Types

- Variable

## Epidemiology

- Most common injury is muscular strain or sprain
- Prevalence of back pain in former elite athletes is 29% compared to 44% for nonathletes.
- 1% to 9% prevalence in runners
- 37% prevalence in soccer players
- 32% to 38% prevalence in tennis players
- 27% prevalence in American football players within an 8-year period

## Pathogenesis

- Sports that require compressive loads with flexion and rotation increase the risk of disc degeneration.
- Calcification and osteophytes develop as the body attempts to autostabilize the segment.

## Risk Factors

- Changes in an athlete's training schedule
- Decreased hamstring flexibility
- Impaired lower extremity biomechanics
- Wrestling, weight lifting, and gymnastics
- Muscle imbalance
- There is no specific association between sports and spinal stenosis.

## Clinical Features

- Pain may develop due to a change in the intensity, duration, or technique during play.
- Sudden onset of symptoms; sometimes the onset of pain may follow a change in the normal routine after only a short period of time.

## Natural History

- Axial low back pain may resolve or progressively worsen.

## Diagnosis

### *Differential diagnosis*

- Colorectal and gynecological malignancies
- Degenerative disc disease
- Infection
- Pancreatitis
- Pars interarticularis stress reaction
- Posterior penetrating stomach ulcers
- Radiculopathy
- Renal disease
- Spinal stenosis
- Spondylolisthesis
- Spondylolysis
- Spondylosis

### *History*

- In general, the pain may present as unilateral or bilateral lower back pain with or without a referral pattern.

### *Exam*

- Antalgic gait
- A step-off at adjacent spinous processes may suggest a compression fracture.
- Hip internal and external rotation to screen for underlying intra-articular hip pathology
- Beyond age 30 the straight leg raise is found to be less reliable.
- Bilateral loss of the ankle reflexes is often a result of advanced age.
- A sacral stress fracture may be worsened with Patrick's test and pain with hopping on the involved side.
- Abdomen should be palpated to rule out the possibility of an abdominal aortic aneurysm.
- Assess for peripheral vascular disease

### *Testing*

- Lab tests for sacroiliac joint pain may include laboratory studies such as a complete blood count, C-reactive protein, and erythrocyte sedimentation rate.
- X-rays of the lumbosacral spine should be considered in cases of direct trauma, midline pain, or lower back deformity.
- A study of MRIs of asymptomatic athletes aged 41 to 69 years, who were active triathletes or handball players, demonstrated similar degenerative changes compared to the general population.
- Former elite soccer players and weight-lifting athletes demonstrate increased degenerative changes compared with the general population.
- Electrodiagnostic studies can assess for possible nerve root lesions or peripheral neuropathy.

### *Pitfalls*

- Only 15% of mature athletes with back pain have a precise pathoanatomical diagnosis.

## Red Flags

- Radiculopathy
- Fracture
- Bowel or bladder dysfunction

## Treatment

### *Medical*

- Short-term NSAIDs
- Muscle relaxants
- Analgesics
- Bracing for spondylolysis
- Acupuncture has been described as helpful.

### *Exercises*

- General strengthening and stretching with emphasis on core abdominal strengthening
- Dynamic stabilization exercises targeting the transverse abdominus and multifidi muscles
- Sports specific exercises and plyometrics

### *Modalities*

- Heat, cold, ultrasound, and transcutaneous electrical nerve stimulation have been used for symptomatic relief of pain and muscle spasms.

### *Injection*

- Trigger point injections for symptoms of myofascial pain
- Medial branch blocks/radiofrequency neurotomy for zygapophyseal (facet) joint–mediated pain
- Epidural steroid injection for radicular symptoms

### *Surgical*

- Dependent on injury or chronicity

### *Consults*

- Physical medicine and rehabilitation
- Neurological or orthopedic-spine surgery

### *Complications of treatment*

- Variable

## Prognosis

- In most athletes the pain is self-limiting.
- Compression fractures are generally stable if only the anterior column is disrupted with >20 degrees of kyphosis.
  - Athlete may return to noncontact sport when they are painfree and may fully return once the fracture has healed in about 6 to 8 weeks.
- Athletes with mild to moderate spinal stenosis may safely return to activity with a program of core strengthening exercises.
- A surgical approach at one level may also allow full return to sport.
- Multilevel surgical treatment may limit or prevent return to sports activities due to adjacent level degeneration.

## Helpful Hints

- Athletes should be instructed to listen to their bodies.

## Suggested Reading

Hackley DR, Wiesel SW. The lumbar spine in the aging athlete. *Clin Sports Med.* 1993;12(3):465–468.

# Back Pain in the Older Population

## Description
Back pain that occurs in the older population

## Etiology/Types
- Variable

## Epidemiology
- Back pain correlates with functional deficits, future disability, and the perception of ease in performing activities of daily living.
- One-year prevalence of back pain is about 31.5% in persons aged 65 years and older.
- 18% to 34% of individuals aged 70 years or older report functional limitations related to back pain.
- Reported back pain is higher among women than among men, possibly related to an increased risk of osteoporosis and vertebral compression fractures and complaining being more socially acceptable than in men.
- Prevalence of back pain decreases at 85 years of age in women and 90 years in men; possibly related to memory deficits, decreased physical activity, and the overshadowing of other medical problems.

## Pathogenesis
- Progressive degenerative cascade as described by Kirkaldy–Willis

## Risk Factors
- Deconditioning related to acute or chronic illness
- Decreased lower extremity strength
- Genetics only mildly influences the development of back pain in older twins.
- Increased depressive symptoms
- Osteoporosis
- Smoking

## Clinical Features
- Axial lower back pain
- Decreased lumbar flexion and extension
- Loss of lumbar lordosis
- 95.5% demonstrate myofascial pain.
- 83.6% demonstrate sacroiliac joint pain.
- 48% demonstrate hip pain.
- 19% demonstrate tender points that correlate with fibromyalgia.
- 26% demonstrate lumbar spinal stenosis.

## Natural History
- Progressive axial low back pain

## Diagnosis

### *Differential diagnosis*
- Central spinal stenosis
- Degenerative disc disease
- Fracture
- Herniated nucleus pulposus
- Myofascial pain
- Neoplasm or metastasis
- Radiculopathy
- Spinal stenosis
- Spondylolisthesis
- Trochanteric bursitis
- Zygapophyseal (facet) joint–mediated pain

### *History*
- Axial lower back pain
- Improvement with recumbency
- Worsened with activity

### *Exam*
- Decreased lumbar flexion and extension
- Thoracic kyphosis
- Loss of lumbar lordosis
- Paraspinal muscle spasm may be associated with an underlying vertebral body compression fracture.
- Patient's ability to roll over gives a good indication of their baseline functional mobility.
- Often tenderness is noted in the gluteus medius and trochanteric region.

### *Testing*
- X-rays are useful for the assessment of vertebral body compression fracture.
- MRI is useful to assess for underlying soft tissue abnormalities and neoplasms.
- With increasing age, abnormal findings increase on imaging studies.

### *Pitfalls*
- Difficulty correlating clinical diagnosis with imaging findings

## Red Flags
- Radiculopathy
- Fracture

- Bowel or bladder dysfunction
- Infection
- Neoplasm

## Treatment

### *Medical*

- Females are more likely to use pain medication
- Short-term NSAIDs
- Muscle relaxants
- Analgesics, although caution should be taken with cognitive changes.
- Caution with pain medications as they may interact with other prescription medications
- Acupuncture has been described to be helpful.
- Long-term pain management may be required to maintain functional mobility.

### *Exercises*

- Focus on treating leg-length discrepancy, poor posture, or poor body mechanics
- Moderate physical activity
- "McKenzie" style mechanical evaluation to determine a direction of preference
- With osteoporosis, there may be restrictions on the degree of overpressure and manual techniques that can be applied.

### *Modalities*

- Heat, cold, ultrasound, and transcutaneous electrical nerve stimulation have been used for symptomatic relief of pain and muscle spasms.

### *Injection*

- Trigger point injections for symptoms of myofascial pain
- Zygapophyseal (facet) joint injections
- Medial branch blocks/radiofrequency neurotomy
- Epidural steroid injection for radicular symptoms

### *Surgical*

- Decompressive surgery may be indicated for spinal stenosis.
- Percutaneous vertebral augmentation may be indicated for unrelenting pain from a vertebral body compression fracture.

### *Consults*

- Physical medicine and rehabilitation
- Neurological or orthopedic-spine surgery
- Pain management
- Geriatrics

### *Complications of treatment*

- Variable

## Prognosis

- Prognosis is based on the underlying pathology.

## Helpful Hints

- Older adults should participate in regular moderate aerobic physical activity, strength, and flexibility training.

## Suggested Reading

Hartvigsen J, Christensen K. Active lifestyle protects against incident low back pain in seniors: a population-based 2-year prospective study of 1387 Danish twins aged 70–100 years. *Spine.* 2007;32(1):76–81.

# Back Pain in Young Athletes

## Description

Back pain that occurs in younger athletes

## Etiology/Types

- Spondylolytic lesions
- Lordotic back pain
- Muscle strain or sprain

## Epidemiology

- In athletes under 12 years of age, a pathologic spondylolytic lesion is noted in up to 50% of cases.
- Prevalence of back pain in the adolescent athlete is 46% compared to the age-matched nonathlete, which is 18%.
- 47% of adolescent low back pain is related to spondylolysis compared to 5% of the adult population.
- Lordotic back pain is the second most common cause of back pain in the adolescent athlete.

## Pathogenesis

- Spondylolysis is most commonly unilateral affecting the L5–S1 segment followed by the L4–L5 segment.
- Low-level repetitive stresses or forceful extension with rotation can fracture the pars interarticularis, irrespective of an inciting event.
- Spondylolisthesis occurs due to a pars interarticularis defect or elongation and can progress during the preadolescent growth spurt.
- Lordotic back pain occurs as the growth spurt continues elongating the axial spine, resulting in tightening the thoracolumbar fascia.
  - Tissue tightness causes a traction apophysitis at the iliac crest or spinous process and may also impinge the adjacent spinous processes resulting in a pseudoarthrosis.

## Risk Factors

- Spondylotic lesions—family history, Alaska natives, repetitive hyperextension in sports such as dance, gymnastics, football, and figure skating

## Clinical Features

- Low back pain of intermittent episodes and of increased severity
- The pain of a spinous process fracture is usually worse than a muscle spasm.
- Lordotic back pain and muscle strain or sprain is a diagnosis of exclusion.

## Natural History

- Variable

## Diagnosis

### *Differential diagnosis*

- Abdominal or genitourinary pathology
- Ankylosing spondylitis
- Apophyseal ring fractures
- Disciitis
- Herniated nucleus pulposus
- Juvenile rheumatoid arthritis
- Lymphoma
- Neuroblastoma
- Osteosarcoma
- Psychogenic low back pain
- Scheuermann's kyphosis
- Spinous process fractures
- Spondylolysis or spondylolisthesis
- Vertebral osteomyelitis

### *History*

- Variable

### *Exam*

- Gait assessment should include heel and toe walking
  - Trendelenburg gait
- Assess for scoliosis, kyphosis, or pelvic obliquity
- Hamstring tightness may manifest with a stiff-legged gait with a short stride
- Step-off deformity if the spondylolisthesis is severe.
- Pars interarticularis defect will cause pain with an ipsilateral one-legged hyperextension test.
- Hyperlordosis of the lumbar spine may be present.

### *Testing*

- Oblique X-rays may demonstrate a pars interarticularis fracture.
- MRI is considered for herniated nucleus pulposes, disciitis, vertebral osteomyelitis and bone marrow edema which is an early sign of a pars interarticularis stress reaction.
- SPECT is the most sensitive test to detect spondylolysis.

### *Pitfalls*

- Parent's expectations on the child's athletic ability and future athletic goals could impair good judgment.

## Red Flags

- Systemic illness
- Radiculopathy
- Fracture
- Bowel or bladder dysfunction
- Neoplasm

## Treatment

### *Medical*

- General approach is to stop the activity for 5 to 7 days with gradual return to activity as the pain subsides.
- Treatment for spondylolysis includes activity modification and rest.
  - An antilordotic brace can be used for immobilization in the acute presentation with a 75% healing rate for early defects.
- Treatment for hyperlordosis targets mobilization of the thoracolumbar spine, hamstrings, and pelvis; may also consider relative rest or the use of antilordotic bracing.

### *Exercises*

- General strengthening and stretching with emphasis on core abdominal strengthening
- Dynamic stabilization exercises targeting the transverse abdominus and multifidi muscles
- Sports specific training

### *Modalities*

- Heat, cold, ultrasound, and transcutaneous electrical nerve stimulation have been used for symptomatic relief of pain and muscle spasms.

### *Injection*

- Trigger point injections for symptoms of myofascial pain

### *Surgical*

- Fusion is considered in patients who have continued pain, progression of slippage, neurologic deficits, or a spondylolisthesis of greater than 50%.

### *Consults*

- Physical medicine and rehabilitation
- Neurologic or orthopedic-spine surgery
- Pediatrics

### *Complications of treatment*

- Complications related to surgery

## Prognosis

- The athlete may return to sports, once pain free and range of motion and strength have return to their preinjury baseline.
- Contact sports are restricted if spondylolisthesis progresses.

## Helpful Hints

- Important to balance current athletic performance with future risk of disability

## Suggested Reading

Sassmannshausen G, Smith BG. Back pain in the young athlete. *Clin Sports Med.* 2002;21(1):121–132.

# Brown-Séquard Syndrome

## Description

Charles Edouard Brown-Séquard in 1849 first described a lateral hemisection of the spinal cord affecting the ascending and descending tracts.

## Etiology/Types

- Due to compression of the corticospinal tracts resulting in ipsilateral motor, proprioception and vibratory sense deficits, and contralateral pain and temperature sensation deficits
- Traditionally associated with knife injuries
- Limited number of pure presentations
- Brown-Séquard plus syndrome is more common and is often mislabeled as a true Brown-Séquard syndrome.
  - Described as an asymmetric paresis with hypalgesia, more pronounced on the less paretic side
  - Both extremities may be paretic

## Epidemiology

- Accounts for 1% to 4% of all traumatic spinal cord injuries (of which there are 11,000 new cases per year) or 40 new cases per million population in the United States
- Average age of injury is 40 years of age.

## Pathogenesis

- The corticospinal motor fibers cross at the junction of the medulla and spinal cord.
  - Ascending sensation and vibratory sense fibers found in the dorsal columns remain ipsilateral to the site of entry and then cross over in the medulla.
- The spinothalamic tract crosses the midline of the cord one to two segments rostral to the entry level so deficits in pain and temperature usually manifest a few levels below the level of injury.
- Loss of ipsilateral autonomic function may also result in a Horner's syndrome.

## Risk Factors

- Blunt trauma
- Cardiac surgery
- Cervical disc herniations from C2–C3 to C6–C7
- Cervical fracture or dislocation related to a fall or motor vehicle accident
- Epidural hematoma
- Extramedullary tumors of the spinal cord
- Gun shot wound
- Intravenous drug use
- Knife wound
- Local radiation
- Primary or metastatic tumor
- Spinal cord herniation
- Thoracic aortic surgery
- Transverse myelitis
- Tuberculosis
- Vertebral artery dissection

## Clinical Features

- Acute or gradual onset of symptoms
- Hemiparesis or hemiparalysis with sensory changes
- Parasthesias

## Natural History

- Acute or gradual onset
- Complete or incomplete presentation

## Diagnosis

### *Differential diagnosis*

- Acute poliomyelitis
- Cervical disc herniation
- Guillain-Barré syndrome
- Multiple sclerosis
- Post-traumatic syringomyelia

### *History*

- Injury
- Hemiparesis or hemiparalysis with sensory changes

### *Exam*

- Findings based on the American Spinal Injury Association (ASIA) impairment scale

### *Testing*

- X-rays are used to assess acute traumatic etiology.
- Magnetic resonance imaging (MRI) is useful in assessing damaged soft tissue structures.

### *Pitfalls*

- Incorrect SCI diagnosis

## Red Flags

- Progressive neurological decline
- Bowel and bladder dysfunction

## Treatment

### Medical

- Symptomatic treatment

### Exercises

- Strengthening and conditioning
- Mobility and activities of daily living training

### Modalities

- Heat, cold, ultrasound, and transcutaneous electrical nerve stimulation have been used for symptomatic relief of pain and muscle spasms.

### Injection

- None

### Surgical

- Anterior decompression may provide the safest route in removing intradural disc fragments with the least amount of spinal cord manipulation to allow for improved recovery.

### Consults

- Physical medicine and rehabilitation
- Neurologic or orthopedic-spine surgery
- Neurology

### Complications of treatment

- Progressive spinal cord injury with symptom deterioration
- Complications related to surgery

## Prognosis

- Best prognosis for walking of all spinal cord injuries
- Complete recovery from Brown-Séquard syndrome following an acute cervical disc herniation was noted in a meta-analysis in 10 of 19 extradural cases versus 3 of 10 intradural cases.
- 75% to 90% of patients are able to ambulate independently on discharge from acute rehabilitation.
- If the upper limb is weaker than the lower limb, patients are more likely to ambulate on discharge.
  - In a series of 38 patients published in 1991, patients spent an average of 35 days in acute care and 79 days in intensive rehabilitation. Of these patients, all improved their functional abilities and 29 patients were able to walk independently, 34 had spontaneous bladder emptying, 36 discharged home, 14 were eventually reemployed.

## Helpful Hints

- For manifestations related to a cervical disc herniation, prompt evaluation and surgical decompression is important.

## Suggested Readings

McKinley W, Santos K, Meade M, Brooke K. Incidence and outcomes of spinal cord injury clinical syndromes. *J Spinal Cord Med.* 2007;30(3):215–224.

Roth EJ, Park T, Pang T, Yarkony GM, Lee MY. Traumatic cervical Brown-Séquard and Brown-Séquard-plus syndromes: the spectrum of presentations and outcomes. *Paraplegia.* 1991;29(9):582–589.

# Cauda Equina Syndrome

## Description

Cauda equina syndrome results in bowel and bladder dysfunction due to an acute compressive neuropathy of the lumbar and sacral nerve roots.

## Etiology/Types

- Trauma
- Central disc protrusion
- Intradural and extradural metastasis
- Ependymomas
- Schwannomas
- Neurilemmoma
- Chiropractic manipulation
- Inadequate surgical decompression
- Nerve root swelling
- Retained disc fragments
- Hematoma
- Vascular insufficiency

## Epidemiology

- Overall incidence in the literature is 1% to 5% of spinal pathology.
- 2% to 6% of lumbar disc herniations can result in cauda equina syndrome.
- Most common in men in the fourth or fifth decade of life
- The L4–L5 level is the most commonly involved site followed by the L5–S1 and L3–L4 levels.

## Pathogenesis

- The cauda equina consists of the conus medullaris, filum terminale, and motor and sensory nerve roots within the spinal canal.
- The conus medullaris terminates between the T12 and L2 levels.
- The nerves supply motor and sensory innervation to the lower extremities and sensation to the perineum, genitalia, and the viscera in the pelvis.
- Cauda equina syndrome results in a flaccid neurogenic bladder and flaccid external anal sphincter, resulting in overflow incontinence of urine and stool as well as loss of genital sensation, erection, and ejaculation.

## Risk Factors

- Lumbar disc herniation
- Trauma

## Clinical Features

- Typically characterized by low back pain, sciatica, saddle and perineal anesthesia, loss of anal tone, loss of bowel or bladder function, and diminished or absent ankle, knee, or bulbocavernous reflexes

## Natural History

- Symptoms may develop within several hours or over a longer period of time.

## Diagnosis

### *Differential diagnosis*

- Conus medullaris syndrome
- Herniated nucleus pulposus
- Lumbar muscle spasm

### *History*

- Deficits with bladder dysfunction are more common than bowel dysfunction.
- Bladder dysfunction may manifest as overflow incontinence, incomplete bladder emptying, or marked bladder distension.
- Gait dysfunction

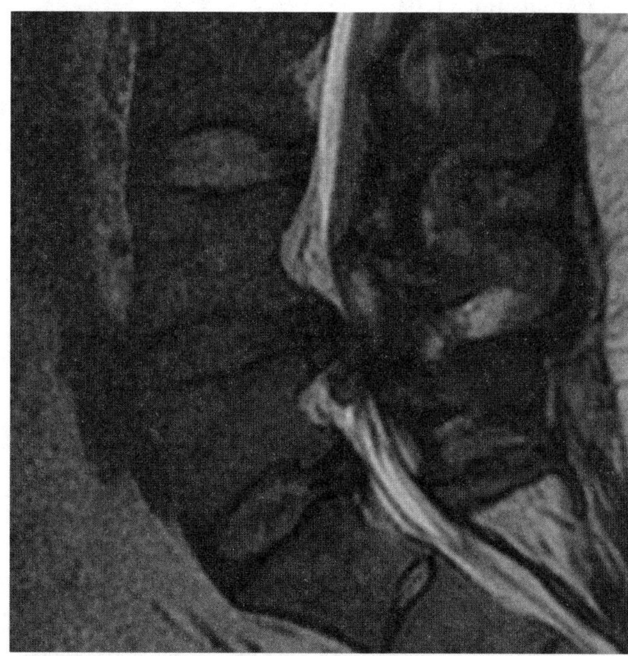

Sagittal lumbar T2-weighted magnetic resonance image demonstrating a large L4–L5 herniated nucleus pulposus that resulted in a cauda equina syndrome. (Courtesy of Keith Hentel, MD.)

### Exam

- Bilateral sciatica or severe bilateral foot weakness with the inability to stand or walk
- Numbness of the perineal region
- Decreased or loss of rectal tone

### Testing

- MRI or CT may demonstrate a large disc extrusion filling up greater than one third of the central canal diameter.

### Pitfalls

- Sometimes it can be difficult to differentiate between an acute foot drop and a chronic radiculopathy that yields a true cauda equina syndrome.

## Red Flags

- Bowel and bladder dysfunction

## Treatment

### Medical

- Preoperative dexamethasone

### Exercises

- Postoperative strengthening and stretching
- Postoperative mobility and activities of daily living training

### Modalities

- Heat, cold, ultrasound, and transcutaneous electrical nerve stimulation have been used for symptomatic relief of pain and muscle spasms.

### Injection

- None

### Surgical

- The goal is decompression within 24 hours
- Laminectomy and discectomy

### Consults

- Neurologic or orthopedic-spine surgery
- Physical medicine and rehabilitation

### Complications of treatment

- Continued bowel, bladder, and motor dysfunction
- Complications related to surgery

## Prognosis

- Prognosis is greatly influenced by the preoperative neurologic state.
- Surgery within 24 hours allows patients to progress from motor strength of 0–1/5 to 4/5 during the postoperative period.
  - Patients are normal or near normal within 6 months to 1 year.
- With delayed surgery, 58% of patients will have persistent motor deficits.
- Motor recovery progresses up to one year
- With emergent surgery, three-fourths of patients were discharged from the hospital on intermittent catheterization. By 6 months 95% of patients who underwent emergent surgery had recovered bladder function.

## Helpful Hints

- Immediate surgical consultation with a goal of decompression within 24 hours

## Suggested Readings

Kennedy JG, Soffe KE, McGrath A, Stephens MM, Walsh MG, McManus F. Predictors of outcome in cauda equina syndrome. *Eur Spine J.* 1999;8(4):317–322.

Shapiro S. Medical realities of cauda equina syndrome secondary to lumbar disc herniation. *Spine.* 2000;25(3):348–351.

# Central Cord Syndrome

## Description

Central cord syndrome was first described by Richard C. Schneider in 1954 as a motor impairment affecting the upper extremities greater than the lower extremities and variable sensory loss below the level of the lesion.

## Etiology/Types

- Sudden compression of the cervical spinal cord between the anterior spondylotic disc-osteophyte complex and the thickened posterior ligamentum flavum with hyperextension of the cervical spine in the older population
- Severe cervical spine trauma in the younger age group
- Acute cervical disc herniations

## Epidemiology

- Age ranges from 18 to 85 years

## Pathogenesis

- Disruption of the medial lamina of the cortical spinal tracts in the central portion of the spinal cord that is responsible for upper-extremity and hand function.
- Sparing of the lateral tracts that are responsible for lower-extremity function.

## Risk Factors

- Diving injuries
- Falls
- Motor vehicle accidents

## Clinical Features

- Presentations vary greatly from minor spinal cord trauma that quickly improves with full neurologic recovery to major spinal cord trauma with significant mortality.
- Bladder dysfunction

## Natural History

- Improvement or worsening of symptoms

## Diagnosis

### *Differential diagnosis*

- Herniated nucleus pulposus
- Other forms of spinal cord injury

### *History*

- History of trauma, fall, or cervical disc herniation

### *Exam*

- Upper-extremity weakness
- Bladder dysfunction
- Variable sensory loss below the level of the lesion

### *Testing*

- MRI can demonstrate increased T2-weighted signal associated with posterior ligamentous injury.
- MRI demonstrates hyperintense signal within the parenchyma of the spinal cord at the level of injury.

### *Pitfalls*

- Up to 24% of central cord syndrome injuries progress to chronic central cord syndrome, characterized by the delayed development of worsening neurological symptoms, including spasticity.

## Red Flags

- Progressive neurologic decline

## Treatment

### *Medical*

- Symptomatic treatment

### *Exercises*

- Strengthening and conditioning
- Mobility and activities of daily living training

### *Modalities*

- Heat, cold, ultrasound, and transcutaneous electrical nerve stimulation have been used for symptomatic relief of pain and muscle spasms.

### *Injection*

- None

### *Surgical*

- Surgical intervention is not required unless there is spinal instability
- Decompressive surgery even after a prolonged nonoperative period may allow for significant improvement if the cause is related to a spondylotic ridge or herniated disc.

### *Consults*

- Neurologic or orthopedic-spine surgery
- Physical medicine and rehabilitation

### *Complications of treatment*

- Considerable recovery can be achieved using a non-surgical approach although a progressive neurologic decline following recovery and plateau has been noted, which is thought to be due to continued spinal cord compression.

- Complications related to surgery

## Prognosis

- Poorer neurologic outcomes correlate with a greater degree of central cervical stenosis.
- Cord hemorrhage correlates with a more severe injury and limited neurologic recovery.
- A more favorable outcome is related to a younger age at presentation and no involvement of the lower extremities.
- Recovery has been described as occurring with motor recovery in the lower extremities followed by improved bladder function. Upper-extremity motor improvement follows next with final improvement in the hands. The return of sensory function does not follow any specific pattern.
- From 1956 to 1965, out of a total of 42 cases: at discharge, 57% patients were functionally ambulatory and 23% were not ambulatory.

## Helpful Hints

- Recovery may continue even after discharge, so it is important to continue intensive outpatient rehabilitation.
- Spasticity influences the ability to ambulate.

## Suggested Readings

Harrop JS, Sharan A, Ratliff J. Central cord injury: pathophysiology, management, and outcomes. *Spine J.* 2006;6 (6 Suppl):198S–206S.

Roth EJ, Lawler MH, Yarkony GM. Traumatic central cord syndrome: clinical features and functional outcomes. *Arch Phys Med Rehabil.* 1990;71(1):18–23.

# Chondrosarcoma

## Description

Chondrosarcoma is a malignant tumor that is made up of a hyaline cartilage matrix and chondrocytes.

## Etiology/Types

- Unknown

## Epidemiology

- Third most common malignant neoplasm after multiple myeloma and osteogenic sarcoma
- Primarily affects the pelvic and shoulder girdle and is very rare in the axial spine.
- 9% of patients have lesions affecting the axial spine, of which 50% affect the lumbosacral spine, followed by 32% at the thoracic spine, and 18% at the cervical spine.
- Usual age of onset ranges from 40 to 60 years.
- Male predominance

## Pathogenesis

- Locally aggressive tumor with limited metastatic capability
- Tumor grows extremely slowly resulting in painless lesions.
- It may grow to a very large size, especially in the pelvis.

## Risk Factors

- Fibrous dysplasia
- Irradiation
- Paget's disease
- Preexisting osteochondroma

## Clinical Features

- May present with mild discomfort or pain and a localized palpable swelling
- Neurologic changes may be the first symptom.
- Up to 50% of patients have neurologic symptoms.

## Natural History

- Tumor grows extremely slowly

## Diagnosis

### *Differential diagnosis*

- Chordoma
- Giant cell tumor
- Osteogenic sarcoma

### *History*

- Mild discomfort
- Palpable swelling
- Neurologic deficits

### *Exam*

- A myelopathic presentation may also develop with invasion or compression of the spinal canal.
- Rectal examination may be indicated to assess for pelvic or sacral tumors.

### *Testing*

- Laboratory tests include complete blood count, chemistry, and sedimentation rates.
- 75% of patients have an abnormal glucose tolerance test with high insulin levels.
- X-rays demonstrate a well-defined lesion with expansive contours and a fluffy or lobular interior with scalloping of the inner cortex.
- Cortical destruction and soft tissue invasion is a characteristic of aggressive tumors.
- CT and MRI allow for delineation of the tumor boundaries in the soft tissue.
- CT detects the calcification of the tumor matrix and destruction of the cortical bone and is more reliable for assessing cortical outlines of the bone and mineralized matrix.
- MRI allows for delineation of tumor penetration into the bone marrow, soft tissue, and spinal canal.
- MRI demonstrates high signal intensity on T2-weighted images, which is thought to be caused by the high water content of the hyaline cartilage.
- Higher grade lesions demonstrate increased diffuse or nodular contrast enhancement.
- A bone scan may detect metastatic lesions.
- Biopsy confirms the diagnosis.
- Arteriography is useful for detecting major feeding vessels, which can help in surgical planning as well as determining the overall extraosseous involvement.

### *Pitfalls*

- Chondrosarcoma with new onset of pain suggests active growth.

## Red Flags

- Myelopathy

## Treatment

### Medical

- No chemotherapeutic agents have been found to be helpful.

### Exercises

- None

### Modalities

- None

### Injection

- None

### Surgical

- Laminectomy or decompression allows for transient improvement in neurologic symptoms.
- En bloc surgical excision with wide histologic margins without contaminating the site with neoplastic cells offers the best chance for a complete cure, although can be technically difficult.

### Consults

- Neurologic or orthopedic-spine surgery

### Complications of treatment

- Surgical complications from an en bloc excision
- Progressive neurologic dysfunction

## Prognosis

- One study found that 50% of patients with contaminated margins died after local recurrence

## Helpful Hints

- Surgery can be technically difficult, and the extent of the resection impacts the recurrence rate and functional rehabilitation.

## Suggested Readings

Camins MB, Duncan AW, Smith J, Marcove RC. Chondrosarcoma of the spine. *Spine.* 1978;3(3):202–209.

Shives TC, McLeod RA, Unni KK, Schray MF. Chondrosarcoma of the spine. *J Bone Joint Surg Am.* 1989;71(8):1158–1165.

# Chordoma

## Description
Chordoma is a low-grade malignancy arising from the embryonic notochord cells in the spine.

## Etiology/Types
- Unknown

## Epidemiology
- Accounts for 3% to 4% of primary bone tumors
- 50% are found in the sacrococcygeal region.
- 35% occur in the basioccipital region.
- Skull-based presentations occur in adolescents and children.
- Most common in the fifth and sixth decade
- Male to female ratio 2:1

## Pathogenesis
- Physaliphorous cells with glycogen and oxidative enzyme-filled vacuoles of notochord origin are a distinct feature.

## Risk Factors
- Trauma

## Clinical Features
- Vague symptoms due to local compression as the tumor enlarges
- Symptoms related to compression of neural elements and pressure on the pelvic structures
- Referred pain to the hip, groin, knee, or sacroiliac joint
- Night pain
- Pain not relieved with recumbency
- Cervical spine presentation may result in unilateral paresthesias or weakness
- Progressive dyspnea if the tumor is located in the cervicothoracic region.

## Natural History
- Slow, clinical course
- Mainly remains local but may metastasize to the lungs, bone, and liver.

## Diagnosis

### *Differential diagnosis*
- Aneurysmal bone cyst
- Chondrosarcoma
- Giant cell tumor
- Intrasacral cysts
- Metastases
- Multiple myeloma
- Osteoblastoma
- Osteochondroma
- Osteosarcoma
- Teratoma

### *History*
- Vague symptoms due to local compression

### *Exam*
- Cervical spine presentation may result in unilateral paresthesias or weakness
- Sacral presentation may be detected by a rectal examination as a firm, round mass on the posterior wall of the rectum
- Spasticity is noted with high lumbar presentations whereas sacral presentations may present with decreased tone.

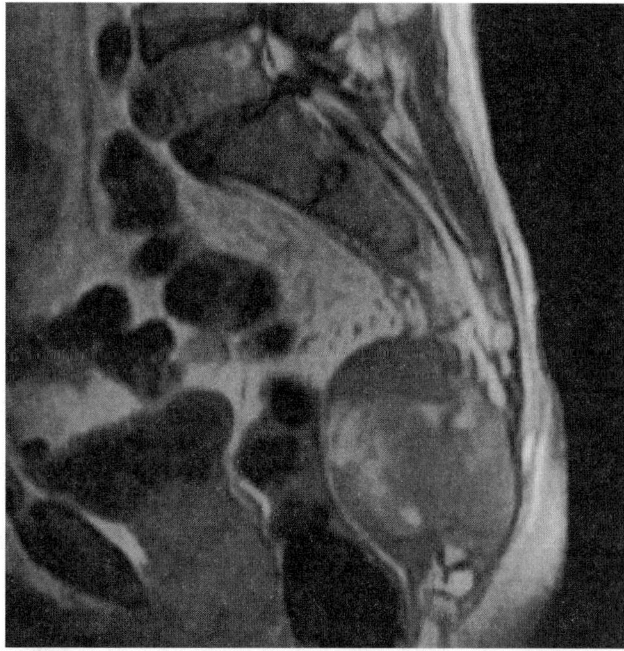

Sagittal lumbosacral T1-weighted magnetic resonance image of a chordoma that has grown into the pelvis, forward displacing the rectum. (Adapted from Fast A, Goldsher D. *Navigating the Adult Spine: Bridging Clinical Practice and Neuroradiology*. New York: Demos Medical Publishing, 2007:111.)

### Testing

- The tumor appears as a well-encapsulated, lobulated, soft grayish mass on gross examination.
- X-rays demonstrate destruction of several segments of the axial or sacral spine with a characteristic appearance of a soft tissue mass with lytic bony destruction and calcified foci.
- A bone scan usually does not show increased uptake at the site.
- CT scan can demonstrate the extent of bony involvement.
- Myelography may miss a sacral presentation as the sacral canal ends at the S2 level
- MRI is useful in staging and diagnosing these lesions based on increased T2-weighted signal compared to the adjacent soft tissues.
- Biopsy is used for definitive diagnosis.
- Sacral chordomas frequently require an open biopsy.

### Pitfalls

- Diagnosis is usually late

## Red Flags

- Progressive dyspnea
- Unstable spine

## Treatment

### Medical

- Radiation therapy is indicated if a complete excision cannot be done and it may slow tumor growth and increase the survival rate.
- Local control at 5 years with proton beam radiation therapy is 50% to 60%.

### Exercises

- None

### Modalities

- None

### Injection

- None

### Surgical

- En bloc excision or high sacral amputation is the preferred method of treatment, although the patient may lose normal bowel and bladder function.
- Tumor spillage may increase the local recurrence rate from 28% to 64%.
- Surgery is limited by technical constraints and quality of life issues.

### Consults

- Neurologic or orthopedic-spine surgery
- Physical medicine and rehabilitation

### Complications of treatment

- Sacral resections above the S2 level result in significant perioperative morbidity and long-term problems.
- Surgical complications from an en bloc excision

## Prognosis

- Prognosis should be based on location, pathology, and invasiveness.
- 5-year survival rates have been reported to be 86% with local recurrence free survival of 60%.
- Local failure rate with a marginal resection can be greater than 70%.

## Helpful Hints

- Local recurrences are frequent
- En bloc excision or high sacral amputation is the preferred method of treatment.

## Suggested Readings

Casali PG, Stacchiotti S, Sangalli C, Olmi P, Gronchi A. Chordoma. *Curr Opin Oncol.* 2007;19(4):367–370.

York JE, Kaczaraj A, Abi-Said D, et al. Sacral chordoma: 40-year experience at a major cancer center. *Neurosurgery.* 1999;44(1):74–79; discussion 79–80.

# Coccydynia (Coccygodynia)

## Description

Coccydynia is pain due to an injury of or originating from the coccyx.

## Etiology/Types

- Associated with obesity, which decreases pelvic rotation with sitting
- Trauma, including falls
- Challenging vaginal delivery that results in subluxation

## Epidemiology

- Mean age of onset is 40 years
- Female to male ratio of 5:1

## Pathogenesis

- Sacrum consists of five fused sacral bones followed by the coccyx, which is a triangular structure made up of three to four fused coccygeal vertebrae.
- Sacral cornu (S5), articulates with the coccygeal cornu via a zygapophyseal (facet) joint disc complex, which can be a symphysis or a synovial joint.
- Coccyx also provides anchor points for the origin of the coccygeal and gluteus maximus muscles as well as the anococcygeal ligaments.
- Mobility of the segments and their angulation do not appear to increase the risk of pain.

## Risk Factors

- Immobile coccyx may result in the formation of a bursitis at the tip.
- Obesity

## Clinical Features

- History of a fall or chronic insidious pain in the buttock
- Worsened with sitting or arising from a seated position, bowel movements, or walking
- Improved with offloading the coccygeal area by shifting weight on either buttock or onto the legs
- Point tenderness at the sacrococcygeal region with associated muscle spasm on rectal examination

## Natural History

- Episodic or continuous, unrelenting, mild to debilitating pain

## Diagnosis

### Differential diagnosis

- Arachnoiditis
- Coccyx and sacral tumors
- Coccyx dislocation or fracture
- Lumbar intervertebral disc disease
- Perirectal abscesses
- Pilonidal cysts
- Posttraumatic arthritis of the sacrococcygeal joint

### History

- History of a fall or worsening buttock pain

### Exam

- Assess for bruising or erythema related to acute trauma
- Assess for pilonidal cysts or fistulas
- Point tenderness at the sacrococcygeal region or the location of trauma
- No tenderness in the adjacent musculature or soft tissue
- Palpate for edema, masses, or bony spicules in the surrounding tissue or intrarectally
- Decreased, increased, or normal coccygeal flexibility
- Reproduction of pain with coccygeal motion
- Intrarectal manipulation may demonstrate similar findings with adjacent musculature muscle spasm.

### Testing

- Lateral X-rays of the coccyx with normal sitting and standing demonstrates a coccygeal pivot of 5 to 25 degrees anteriorly or posteriorly with sitting, returning to the normal position with standing.
- Coccyx in symptomatic patients pivots anteriorly >25 degrees or subluxes posteriorly with sitting.
- MRI may demonstrate increased T2 signal at the hypermobile or subluxed segment.
- Technetium Tc-99m bone scan may demonstrate increased activity at the hypermobile or subluxed segment.

### Pitfalls

- Often takes years for a firm diagnosis
- May impact academic or vocational performance
- Acute presentations may be very debilitating

## Red Flags

- Important to rule out a metastasis or tumor if the patient notes blood during defecation

## Treatment

### Medical

- Short-term NSAIDs
- Muscle relaxants
- Analgesics
- Hot baths
- Cushion

### Exercises

- Pelvic floor strengthening especially following pregnancy

### Modalities

- 16% of patients improved with 2 weeks of ultrasound followed by 2 weeks of diathermy.
- Manipulation is thought to relax intrapelvic muscle tension of the levator ani, coccygeus, and piriformis muscles.
- One study demonstrated that three to four sessions of levator anus massage and stretching were more effective than joint mobilization alone, and those patients with an immobile coccyx fared worse than patients with a mobile coccyx.

### Injection

- Diagnostic block with local anesthetic may also be helpful in diagnosing a hypermobile or subluxed segment.
- Steroid infiltration of the sides and tip of the coccyx may be helpful.
- Repeated flexion and extension of the coccyx for one minute under general anesthesia may be helpful.
- Fluoroscopically guided ganglion impar blocks via the sacrococcygeal junction or first intracoccygeal junction

### Surgical

- Surgical indications include disabling coccyx pain with radiographic signs of subluxation, instability, or a bone spur
- Coccygectomy demonstrates a 60% to 91% success rate.

### Consults

- Orthopedic-spine surgery
- Physical medicine and rehabilitation

### Complications of treatment

- Surgical complications include wound infection ranging from 2% to 22%.

## Prognosis

- Good outcomes noted with nonsurgical and surgical treatments.

## Helpful Hints

- Often chronic pain which takes years for a firm diagnosis

## Suggested Readings

Foye PM, Buttaci CJ, Stitik TP, Yonclas PP. Successful injection for coccyx pain. *Am J Phys Med Rehabil.* 2006;85(9):783–784.

Wray CC, Easom S, Hoskinson J. Coccydynia: aetiology and treatment. *J Bone Joint Surg Br.* 1991;73:335–338.

# Deconditioning

## Description

Deconditioning should be considered a separate condition from the original illness.

## Etiology/Types

- Loss of normal physiological load on tissues

## Epidemiology

- Common in hospitalized patients or other situations of significantly decreased activity
- More common in the older population

## Pathogenesis

- Horizontal positioning reduces energy consumption and increases the chances of surviving a medical crisis, but also accelerates the process of deconditioning.
- Peak aerobic capacity can be reduced by up to 31% after 30 days of bed rest.
- The change in $VO_{2max}$ is based on the premorbid level of aerobic conditioning and the duration of bed rest, but is not affected by age or gender.
- The physiological mechanisms responsible for deconditioning include decreased maximal stroke volume and cardiac output; decreased venous return caused by lower blood volume; and decreased pulmonary capacity.
- Muscle weakening is thought to be related to the loss of muscle mass and changes in motor control, contractile properties, electromechanical coupling, and decreased nerve conduction.
- Three weeks of inactivity in the peripheral joints can cause an alteration in tendon stiffness and increase bone turnover, resulting in an increased risk of sprains and fractures during the rehabilitation process
- 9% loss of muscle mass in the multifidus and erector spinae with only a few weeks of horizontal bed rest
- Patients without a history of low back pain who are required to remain in bed for prolonged periods of time may compromise the function of their multifidus muscles, predisposing them to future lower back pain.
- Overall, may lose up to 1% to 1.5% of muscle strength per day.
- Prolonged immobility may result in a loss of 25% to 40% of muscle strength.

## Risk Factors

- Chronic prolonged illness
- Immobility

## Clinical Features

- Based on primary illness and the premorbid level of conditioning
- Significant muscle wasting
- Poor endurance
- Joint contractures
- Loss of strength is greater in the proximal muscles compared with the distal muscles.

## Natural History

- Progressive worsening with decreased activity

## Diagnosis

### *Differential diagnosis*

- Cardiopulmonary disease
- Connective tissue disease
- Critical illness polyneuropathy
- Multiple sclerosis
- Neuropathy
- Steroid myopathy

### *History*

- Generalized weakness
- Decreased endurance

### *Exam*

- Muscle wasting
- Joint contractures
- Difficulty with functional tasks

### *Testing*

- Electrodiagnostic studies may demonstrate decreased motor unit action potentials and/or denervation with severe wasting.

### *Pitfalls*

- Overlooked treatable underlying diagnosis

## Red Flags

- Progressive myopathy or neuropathy

## Treatment

### *Medical*

- Proper nutrition to support muscle development

### *Exercises*

- Patients with 2 weeks of bed rest will not return to their pre–bed rest cardiovascular response even after 3 weeks of ambulation and mild exercise.
- Severe deconditioning requires a period of immobilization three times as long as the initial requirement in order to regain lost strength.
- Minimal daily isometrics exercises can significantly decrease the progression.
- Strengthening and conditioning
- Stretching
- Neuromuscular reeducation and coordination
- Proprioception and balance exercises
- Mobility and activities of daily living training

### *Modalities*

- Heat, cold, ultrasound, and transcutaneous electrical nerve stimulation have been used for symptomatic relief of pain and muscle spasms.

### *Injection*

- None

### *Surgical*

- None

### *Consults*

- Nutrition
- Geriatrics in the older patient population

### *Complications of treatment*

- Muscle strains or sprains
- Tendonopathies
- Pain from reconditioning program
- Increased risk of fracture, especially in osteopenic or osteoporotic patients

## Prognosis

- Generally good to excellent
- Overall based on underlying health status

## Helpful Hints

- Patients have to understand that reconditioning is a long, slow process.

## Suggested Readings

Bloomfield SA. Changes in musculoskeletal structure and function with prolonged bed rest. *Med Sci Sports Exerc.* 1997;29(2):197–206.

Rader MC, Vaughen JL. Management of the frail and deconditioned patient. *South Med J.* 1994;87(5):S61–S65.

# Diffuse Idiopathic Skeletal Hyperostosis (Forrestier's Disease)

## Description

Diffuse idiopathic skeletal hyperostosis (DISH) manifests as axial spine stiffness and pain and is characterized by calcification of the spinal and the adjacent extraspinal structures on plain radiographs.

## Etiology/Types

- Generally unknown etiology
- Possibly related to occupational stress and trauma
- Insulin and retinoic acid may play a role as they may act as bone growth factors

## Epidemiology

- Common in men aged 48 to 85 years
- Male to female ratio is 2:1
- Most common in whites, Asians, and Native Americans
- Found in 6% to 28% of autopsies

## Pathogenesis

- Calcification and ossification occur in soft tissues, particularly the ligaments and entheses.

## Risk Factors

- Unknown

## Clinical Features

- 57% of patients initially complain of thoracolumbar back pain.
- 50% of patients report neck pain.
- 80% of affected individuals complain of spinal stiffness 10 to 20 years before diagnosis.
- Right-sided preference in the axial spine
- Mild to severe dysphagia occurs in 17% to 28% of patients with anterior osteophytes in the cervical spine.
- 37% of patients have extraspinal enthesopathies in the peripatellar ligaments, plantar fascia, olecranon, and the Achilles tendons.
- 50% of patients with DISH also have ossification of the posterior longitudinal ligament (OPLL).
- Associated with ossification of the ligamentum flavum

## Natural History

- Progressive axial spine stiffness and pain
- Potential development of cervical myelopathy, spinal cord injury, and dysphagia

## Diagnosis

### Differential diagnosis

- Acromegaly
- Hypoparathyroidism
- Neuropathic arthropathy
- Ochronosis
- Spondyloarthropathies
- Trauma

### History

- Stiffness improves during the day
- Stiffness worse in the morning and evening
- Stiffness worsens with immobility

### Exam

- Decreased cervical and lumbar lordosis
- Affected extraspinal joints may demonstrate decreased range of motion.
- Normal axial spine range of motion is preserved because the posterior elements do not fuse.

### Testing

- Diagnosis is based on radiographic findings using Resnick and Niwayama's criteria.
- Recognized on X-rays by flowing ossification along the anterolateral vertebrae of at least four contiguous vertebrae with the absence of a spondyloarthropathy or degenerative changes.
- X-ray findings include the absence of sacroiliac joint sclerosis, erosion, or fusion; preservation of disc heights without evidence of degenerative disc disease; absence of apophyseal joint bony ankylosis.
- Thoracic and L1–L3 lumbar involvement are the most common findings.
- C4–C7 segments are the most commonly affected vertebrae in the cervical spine.
- MRI is useful in locating suspected fractures in the vertebral bodies, based on intervertebral fluid collections or assessing for OPLL.

### Pitfalls

- Spinal fractures in older patients may be missed or delayed in diagnosis due to their baseline pain with an increased risk of neurologic sequelae with spinal instability.

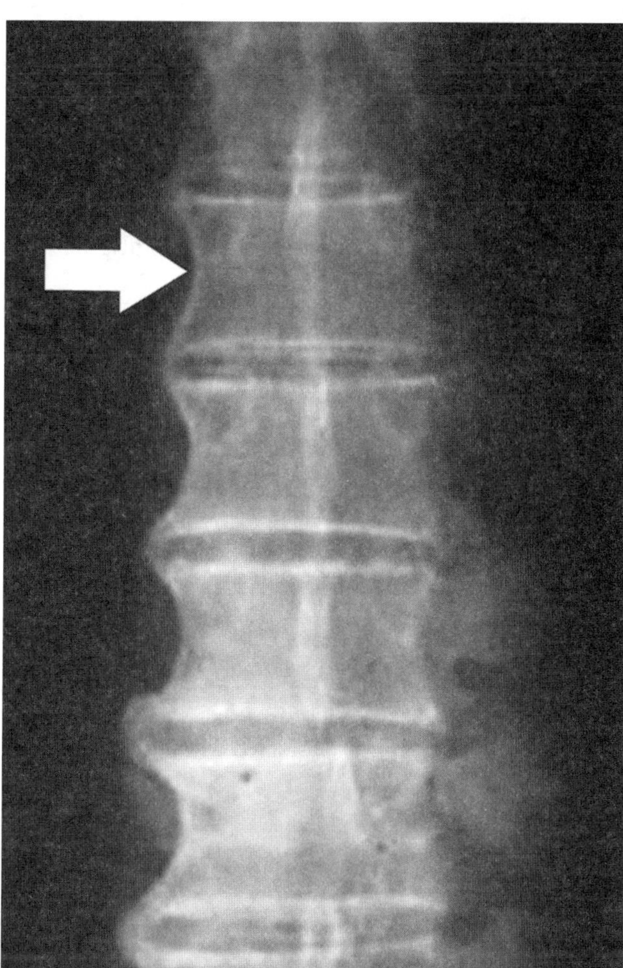

Anterioposterior AP thoracic plain radiograph demonstrating flowing osteophytes bridging greater than four vertebral bodies (arrow) in a patient with diffuse idiopathic skeletal hyperostosis. (Adapted from Fast A, Goldsher D. *Navigating the Adult Spine: Bridging Clinical Practice and Neuroradiology.* New York: Demos Medical Publishing, 2007:82.)

## Red Flags

- Neurologic compromise from spinal cord impingement or dysphagia from cervical spine involvement

## Treatment

### *Medical*

- Focus on pain relief and maximizing function
- NSAIDs for pain control

### *Exercises*

- General strengthening and stretching
- Home exercise programs focus on maintaining axial spine flexibility

### *Modalities*

- Heat, cold, ultrasound, and transcutaneous electrical nerve stimulation have been used for symptomatic relief of pain and muscle spasms.

### *Injection*

- Trigger point injections for symptoms of myofascial pain

### *Surgical*

- Surgery may be considered in patients with dysphagia associated with anterior cervical osteophytes although recurrence is possible.

### *Consults*

- Neurologic or orthopedic-spine surgery
- Physical medicine and rehabilitation

### *Complications of treatment*

- Variable

## Prognosis

- Benign course

## Helpful Hints

- Assess for spinal fractures in older patients

## Suggested Reading

Sarzi-Puttini P, Atzeni F. New developments in our understanding of DISH (diffuse idiopathic skeletal hyperostosis). *Curr Opin Rheumatol.* 2004;16(3):287–292.

# Disciitis

## Description

Disciitis is an infection of the intervertebral disc space.

## Etiology/Types

- Osteomyelitis
- Hematogenous spread and direct inoculation during an interventional procedure or surgery

## Epidemiology

- Uncommon in adults
- Reported in patients into the sixth decade
- 2.8% develop an infection following lumbar disc surgery
- Male predominance

## Pathogenesis

- Hematogenous spread is considered the route of entry in children.
- Lumbar spine is affected in 77% of cases, the cervical spine in 15%, and the thoracic spine in 8%.
- Gram-positive organisms include *Staphylococcus aureus*, *Streptococcus epidermidis*, and *Streptococcus milleri*.
- Gram-negative organisms include *Pseudomonas aeruginosa*, *Escherichia coli*, and *Campylobacter fetus*.
- Fungal organisms include *Aspergillus fumigatus*.
- Biopsy specimens may demonstrate cellular necrosis and adjacent vertebral osteomyelitis.

## Risk Factors

- Absent prophylactic antibiotic coverage prior to an invasive procedure
- Adjacent abscess
- Cerebral angiography
- Debilitated patients
- Diabetes
- Discography
- Epidural anesthesia during delivery
- Fracture
- Heavy physical labor
- Immunocompromised patients
- Needle biopsy of the intervertebral disc
- Operative procedures
- Trauma

## Clinical Features

- Localized spinal pain ranging from mild and insidious to acute and severe
- The pain may radiate to the upper extremities and hands if originating from the cervical spine or the abdomen, flanks and lower extremities if originating from the thoracic or lumbar spine.

## Natural History

- Progressively worsening pain and disability over 2 years before a diagnosis is confirmed.

## Diagnosis

### *Differential diagnosis*

- Calcium pyrophosphate dehydrate crystal deposition
- Chordoma
- Degenerative disc disease
- Myeloma
- Osteomyelitis of the vertebral body
- Spinal erosive changes associated with chronic renal failure
- Trauma

### *History*

- Sharp, severe pain
- Pain may be referred to the extremities
- Pain worsens with movement, improved with rest
- A period of postsurgical improvement followed by worsening pain
- Preference for recumbency

### *Exam*

- Fever is rare
- Localized tenderness to palpation
- Limited axial spine range of motion
- Neurologic deficits that suggest myelopathy or spinal cord compression

### *Testing*

- Elevated erythrocyte sedimentation rate, C-reactive protein, and leukocytosis
- Blood cultures may be positive
- Culture of the infectious fluid or tissue may be positive
- Plain radiographs may demonstrate loss of disc height, adjacent reactive sclerosis of the subchondral bone, irregularity of the end plates.
- Bone scan may demonstrate increased bony activity within the adjacent vertebral bodies.
- CT can demonstrate disc space narrowing and erosion through the endplate
- MRI can detect changes before plain radiographs.

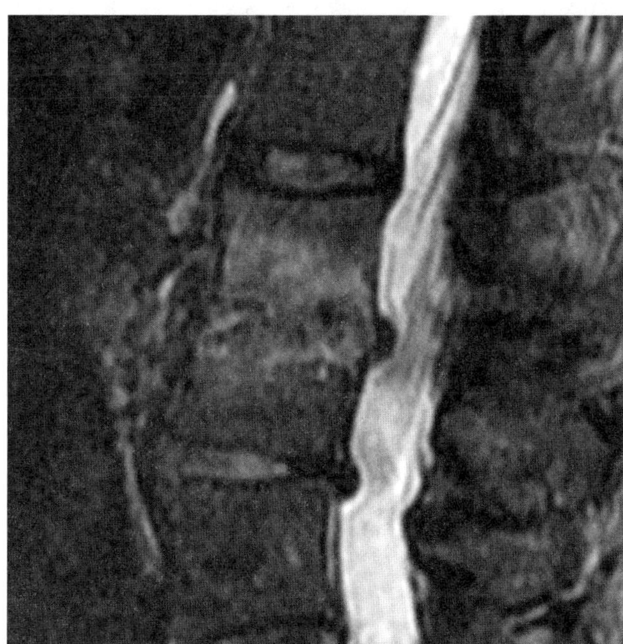

Sagittal lumbar T2-weighted magnetic resonance image with fat suppression demonstrating intervertebral disc destruction and progressive involvement of the adjacent vertebral bodies associated with disciitis. (Courtesy of Keith Hentel, MD.)

### Pitfalls

- Diagnostic delay

## Red Flags

- Associated radiculopathy or paraparesis

## Treatment

### Medical

- A 4- to 6-week course of antibiotics
- Immobilization
- Bracing
- Bed rest

### Exercises

- None

### Modalities

- Modalities are contraindicated as they may increase the spread of the infectious process.

### Injection

- None

### Surgical

- Surgery is reserved for spinal instability, deformity, and cord compression.
- CT-guided percutaneous drainage
- Surgical fusion is usually unnecessary.

### Consults

- Neurologic or orthopedic-spine surgery
- Infectious disease

### Complications of treatment

- Complications related to surgery include hemiplegia and tetraplegia.

## Prognosis

- The prognosis in children is good, as arterioles supply the developing end plates in children.
- Antibiotics given early can limit the extent of intervertebral disc and vertebral body destruction.

## Helpful Hints

- Early identification and treatment is crucial.

## Suggested Reading

Schulitz KP, Assheuer J. Discitis after procedures on the intervertebral disc. *Spine.* 1994;19(10):1172–1177.

# Ehlers–Danlos Syndrome

## Description

Ehlers–Danlos syndrome (EDS) is a rare hereditary collagen metabolism disorder resulting in joint and soft tissue hypermobility.

## Etiology/Types

- Classic
- Hypermobile
- Vascular
- Kyphoscoliosis
- Arthrochalasia
- Dermatosparaxis

## Epidemiology

- Estimated incidence is 1 in 5,000 live births.

## Pathogenesis

- Mutations affect type I and III procollagen or enzymes that modify collagen.
- Defect in the formation of collagen fibrils

## Risk Factors

- Hereditary

## Clinical Features

- Joint hypermobility with possible subluxation or dislocation
- Skin hyperextensibility and fragility
- Friable soft tissues with easy bruising and poor healing
- Kyphoscoliosis is common in type IV EDS.
- Pigmented scars over the bony prominences of the epicanthal folds, forehead, and chin
- Blue sclera
- Wide-set eyes
- Thin cheek bones
- "Lobeless" ears
- Patients may be able to touch the tip of their nose with their tongue
- Weak collapsible handclasp
- Pes planus
- Early osteoarthritis
- Shoulder laxity and instability
- Soft velvety skin
- Poor vision
- Mitral valve prolapse
- Aortic aneurysm
- Obstetric or gynecologic complications
- Increased risk of Chiari I malformation

## Natural History

- Hypermobility causes back pain in 6% to 67% of affected individuals.
- Spinal deformity is most common in the arthrochalasia, kyphoscoliosis, and classic types.
- Spondylosis or spondylolysis may also develop due to tissue laxity.

## Diagnosis

### *Differential diagnosis*

- Marfan syndrome
- Osteogenesis imperfecta
- Other collagen vascular disorders

### *History*

- Back pain
- Kyphoscoliosis

### *Exam*

- Joint hypermobility
- Skin hyperextensibility and fragility
- Friable soft tissues with easy bruising and poor healing
- Hypermobile spine
- Spinal deformity
- Assessed using the Beighton scale (Carter–Wilkinson criteria)

### *Testing*

- Plain radiographs demonstrate kyphoscoliosis at the thoracolumbar junction with anterior wedging and posterior scalloping of the vertebral bodies.

### *Pitfalls*

- Osteoporosis

## Red Flags

- Vascular injuries such as bleeding or compartment syndrome
- Sciatic neuropathy

## Treatment

### *Medical*

- Nonoperative treatment preferred
- Brace trial during adolescent growth stage may prevent the formation of scoliosis.

- Education regarding behavior modifications, proper ergonomics, and posture is very important.

### *Exercises*

- Strengthening and proprioception exercises
- General strengthening and stretching with emphasis on core abdominal strengthening
- Low impact aerobic exercise such as swimming

### *Modalities*

- Heat, cold, ultrasound, and transcutaneous electrical nerve stimulation have been used for symptomatic relief of pain and muscle spasms.

### *Injection*

- Trigger point injections and epidural injections may be done for symptomatic relief and should be done with caution due to vessel friability and poor wound healing potential.

### *Surgical*

- Fusion for progressive spine deformity

### *Consults*

- Physical medicine and rehabilitation
- Rheumatology
- Neurologic or orthopedic-spine surgery for spinal instability

### *Complications of treatment*

- Surgical complications include poor healing potential, wound dehiscence, paraplegia, radiculopathy, vascular injury, and abnormal scar formation due to abnormal tissue resilience.

## Prognosis

- Unknown

## Helpful Hints

- Education regarding behavior modifications, proper ergonomics, and posture is very important.

## Suggested Readings

Akpinar S, Gogus A, Talu U, Hamzaoglu A, Dikici F. Surgical management of the spinal deformity in Ehlers-Danlos syndrome type VI. *Eur Spine J.* 2003;12(2):135–140.

McMaster MJ. Spinal deformity in Ehlers-Danlos syndrome. Five patients treated by spinal fusion. *J Bone Joint Surg Br.* 1994;76(5):773–777.

Schroeder EL, Lavallee ME. Ehlers-Danlos syndrome in athletes. *Curr Sports Med Rep.* 2006;5(6):327–334.

# Epidural Abscess

## Description

An epidural abscess is a rare medical emergency that may result in severe and irreversible neurologic deficits.

## Etiology/Types

- 66% of cases are due to *Staphylococcus aureus.*
- Increasing incidence of methicillin-resistant *S. aureus* (MRSA)
- *Staphylococci epidermidis*
- *Escherichia coli*
- *Pseudomonas aeruginosa*
- Fungi
- Mycobacteria
- Parasites

## Epidemiology

- 1 in 10,000 hospital admissions
- Male predominance

## Pathogenesis

- Contiguous (33%) or hematogenous (50%) spread
- Direct compression or vascular occlusion (septic thrombophlebitis) of the spinal cord
- Usually extends over three to four spinal segments
- Osteomyelitis is associated with 80% of epidural abscesses.

## Risk Factors

- Alcoholism
- Catheter or stimulator placement
- Degenerative joint disease
- Diabetes mellitus
- Epidural analgesia
- HIV
- Increasing age
- Injection-drug use
- Nerve blocks
- Sepsis
- Skin or soft tissue infection
- Spinal instrumentation
- Trauma
- Urinary tract infection

## Clinical Features

- Stage 1: Acute onset, severe neck, or back pain at the affected level (75% of patients)
- Stage 2: Progressive radicular pain
- Stage 3: Motor and sensory dysfunction with bowel and bladder dysfunction (33% of patients)
- Stage 4: Spinal cord compressive injury or infarction resulting in paralysis affects 4% to 22% of patients
- Fever (50% of patients)

## Natural History

- Progressive constitutional illness and back pain with progressive neurologic dysfunction and paralysis leading occasionally to death

## Diagnosis

### *Differential diagnosis*

- Discitis
- Endocarditis
- Osteomyelitis
- Sepsis
- Spinal hematoma
- Transverse myelitis
- Urinary tract infection

### *History*

- Acute onset
- Severe neck or back pain
- Progressive neurologic deficit

### *Exam*

- Disorientation
- Fever
- Progressive neurologic deficit
- Bowel or bladder dysfunction

### *Testing*

- Elevated erythrocyte sedimentation rate, C reactive protein, and leukocytosis
- Bacteremia is present in 60% of cases.
- CSF analysis demonstrates increased protein and pleocytosis.
- X-rays may demonstrate disk space narrowing or bone lysis but is not useful in 20% of cases.
- MRI with intravenous gadolinium contrast
- CT-guided needle aspiration
- Bone scan may show increased uptake.

### *Pitfalls*

- 11% to 75% of cases are misdiagnosed.
- The classic triad of back pain, neurologic dysfunction, and fever is not common.

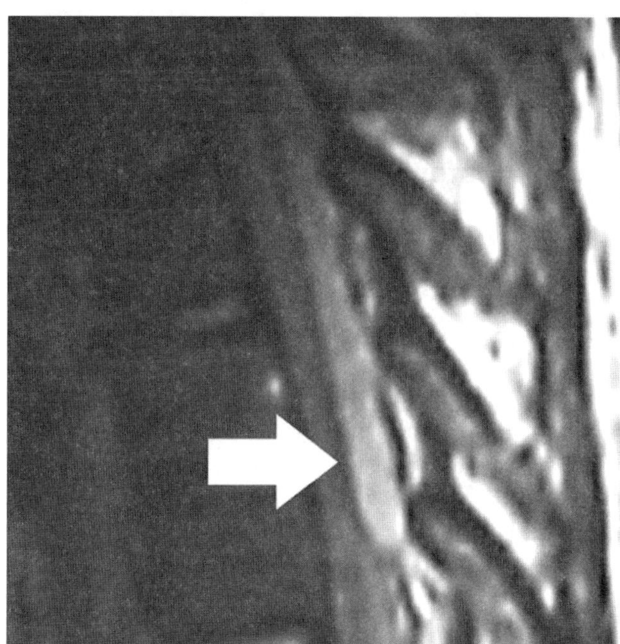

Sagittal thoracic T2-weighted magnetic resonance image demonstrating a hyperintense mass dorsal to the spinal cord (arrow) characteristic of an epidural abscess. (Adapted from Fast A, Goldsher D. *Navigating the Adult Spine: Bridging Clinical Practice and Neuroradiology.* New York: Demos Medical Publishing, 2007:66.)

## Red Flags

- Progressive neurologic decline

## Treatment

### Medical

- Empiric antibiotics against *S. aureus* with vancomycin to cover for MRSA and a third- or fourth-generation cephalosporin to cover for gram-negative bacilli should be used while cultures are pending.
- Systemic antibiotics can be used alone in patients with little or no neurologic compromise, although neurologic compromise can occur with appropriate antibiotics.
- Intravenous antibiotic treatment for 6 weeks due to the coexistence of osteomyelitis

### Exercises

- None

### Modalities

- Modalities are contraindicated as they may increase the spread of the infectious process.

### Injection

- None

### Surgical

- Decompressive laminectomy with debridement is done urgently due to the unknown rate of progression.

### Consults

- Infectious disease
- Neurologic or orthopedic-spine surgery

### Complications of treatment

- Persistent neurologic dysfunction

## Prognosis

- Preoperative neurologic status immediately before surgery is the best predictor of final neurologic outcome.
- Patients with paralysis of >24 to 36 hours may gain some neurologic function up to one year.
- 5% to 16% mortality rate

## Helpful Hints

- The classic triad of back pain, neurologic dysfunction, and fever is not common.

## Suggested Reading

Darouiche RO. Spinal epidural abscess. *N Engl J Med.* 2006;355(19):2012–2020.

# Epidural Lipomatosis

## Description

Epidural lipomatosis is the accumulation of normal fatty tissue in the extradural space encroaching on the spinal canal and compressing the neural elements that results in neurologic dysfunction.

## Etiology/Types

- Unknown

## Epidemiology

- More common in the thoracic spine followed by the lumbar spine
- Never reported in the cervical spine
- Male predominance
- Mean age of onset is 43 years, although it has been described in a 6-year-old undergoing exogenous corticosteroid therapy.

## Pathogenesis

- The spinal cord and nerve roots are slowly compressed.

## Risk Factors

- Asthma
- Anabolic steroid use
- Cushing's disease
- Epidural steroid injections
- Exogenous corticosteroid therapy ranging from 5 to 180 mg per day (most common)
- Hypothyoidism
- Idiopathic
- Inhaled steroids
- Morbid obesity
- Pituitary prolactinoma
- Polyarteritis nodosa
- Radiation pneumonitis
- Renal transplants
- Rheumatoid arthritis

## Clinical Features

- Back pain is the most common symptom.
- Lower-extremity motor and sensory deficits
- Upper or lower motor neuron signs
- Decreased proprioception
- Sphincter dysfunction

## Natural History

- Unknown
- May occur 6 months to 13 years after the beginning of corticosteroid medication

## Diagnosis

### *Differential diagnosis*

- Arteriovenous malformation
- Collagen vascular disease
- Epidural hematoma
- Epidural abscess
- Heavy metal poisoning
- Neoplasm
- Peripheral neuropathy or myopathy related to medication or diabetes
- Porphyria
- Vertebral body compression fracture related to osteoporosis

### *History*

- Back pain

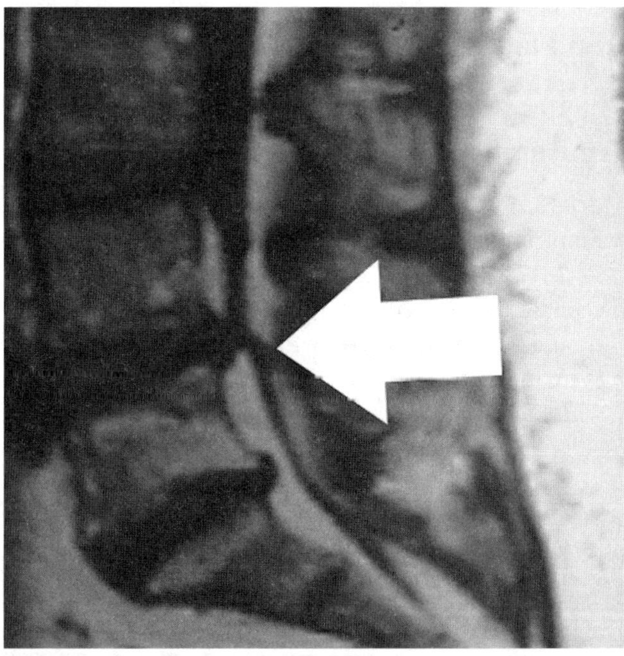

Sagittal lumbar T1-weighted magnetic resonance image demonstrating dural sac compression at L4 and below (arrow) caused by fatty tissue in epidural lipomatosis. (Adapted from Fast A, Goldsher D. *Navigating the Adult Spine: Bridging Clinical Practice and Neuroradiology.* New York: Demos Medical Publishing, 2007:52.)

- Weakness
- Sensory loss
- Burning dysesthesias

### Exam

- Upper or lower motor neuron signs
- Positive straight leg raise

### Testing

- Workup to assess for overproduction of endogenous corticosteroid in idiopathic cases
- MRI demonstrates increased T1-weighted signal and intermediate T2-weighted signal in the lipid mass.
- CT can be used to demonstrate soft tissue surrounding the thecal sac.

### Pitfalls

- Subclinical lumbar stenosis due to degeneration versus epidural lipomatosis in older patients

## Red Flags

- Cauda equina syndrome
- Progressive lower-extremity weakness

## Treatment

### Medical

- Discontinuation of corticosteroid therapy
- Weight reduction in obese patients

### Exercises

- None

### Modalities

- Heat, cold, ultrasound, and transcutaneous electrical nerve stimulation have been used for symptomatic relief of pain and muscle spasms.

### Injection

- None

### Surgical

- Laminectomy with epidural adipose tissue resection is required for cauda equina syndrome or spinal cord compression.

### Consults

- Physical medicine and rehabilitation
- Neurologic or orthopedic spine surgery

### Complications of treatment

- Increased mortality with laminectomies in patients requiring high-dose corticosteroid therapy

## Prognosis

- Epidural fatty tissue may disappear with associated resolution of symptoms following discontinuation of exogenous corticosteroid therapy.
- Outcomes of surgical decompression in the lumbar region tend to be more successful compared to the thoracic region.
- 22% mortality rate within one year in one study due to significant comorbidities in patients who have had laminectomies
- Recurrence of fatty tissue is rare.

## Helpful Hints

- Obese patients may respond to a conservative weight-loss approach.

## Suggested Readings

Fassett DR, Schmidt MH. Spinal epidural lipomatosis: a review of its causes and recommendations for treatment. *Neurosurg Focus.* 2004;16(4):E11.

Fessler RG, Johnson DL, Brown FD, Erickson RK, Reid SA, Kranzler L. Epidural lipomatosis in steroid-treated patients. *Spine.* 1992;17(2):183–188.

Ishikawa Y, Shimada Y, Miyakoshi N, et al. Decompression of idiopathic lumbar epidural lipomatosis: diagnostic magnetic resonance imaging evaluation and review of the literature. *J Neurosurg Spine.* 2006;4(1):24–30.

# Ewing's Sarcoma

## Description

Ewing's sarcoma is a malignant round cell tumor of bone and soft tissue primarily affecting children and adolescents.

## Etiology/Types

- Most cases are characterized by a t(11;22)(q24;q12) balanced translocation.

## Epidemiology

- Second most common malignant primary bone tumor in children and adolescents
- Typical age of presentation is 12 to 24 years.
- Male to female ratio of 2:1
- 3.5% occur in the axial spine
- Most common sites of occurrence are the pelvis, tibia, fibula, and femur.

## Pathogenesis

- Primary malignant sarcoma
- Uniform small blue round cells noted with microscopy
- Grossly it is grayish white and soft.

## Risk Factors

- Unknown

## Clinical Features

- Typically presents as local pain, palpable mass, and neurologic deficits
- Low back pain is usually the first symptom.
- 58% of patients have neurologic deficits.
- Possible overlying point tenderness on the axial spine

## Natural History

- Increased local pain and progressive neurologic deficits

## Diagnosis

### *Differential diagnosis*

- Malignant lymphoma
- Neuroblastoma
- Primitive neuroectodermal tumor of bone
- Rhabdomyosarcoma

### *History*

- Low back pain
- Neurologic dysfunction

### *Exam*

- Palpable mass
- Neurologic deficits

### *Testing*

- Light microscopy
- Immunohistochemical and possibly cytogenetic analysis
- X-rays are normal initially but eventually demonstrate vertebral lytic bone destruction.
- MRI allows for early detection and allows for understanding the extent of soft tissue involvement, including the epidural space and extension into the bone marrow.
- The tumor demonstrates decreased signal on T1-weighted images.
- CT assesses the extent of bony involvement, as well as outlines the extent of soft tissue involvement.
- Large bore needle biopsy should be done rather than an open biopsy through a laminectomy, as this decreases the risk of postlaminectomy kyphosis.
- Bone scan can be used to assess for systemic disease.

### *Pitfalls*

- Progressive neurologic dysfunction

## Red Flags

- Neurologic deficits

## Treatment

### *Medical*

- Radiation
- Chemotherapy regimens include vincristine, actinomycin, and cyclophosphamide with or without adriamycin.

### *Exercises*

- None

### *Modalities*

- None

### *Injection*

- None

### *Surgical*

- En bloc spondylectomy should be considered if there is no evidence of metastasis as long-term survival may be increased.

### *Consults*

- Neurologic or orthopedic-spine surgery

### *Complications of treatment*

- En bloc spondylectomy within the axial spine can be very challenging.
- Radiation-associated sarcoma and myelopathy
- Postlaminectomy kyphosis is the most common complication, which can lead to progressive kyphosis and eventual neurologic compromise.
  - Caused by loss of the posterior tension band following a decompressive laminectomy, which can result in spinal instability.
  - Risk decreased with spinal stabilization

## Prognosis

- Long-term disease-free survival rates with either surgery or radiation ranges from 5% to 20 %, but with chemotherapy along with radiation or surgery the survival rate jumps to 50% to 80%.
- Recurrence rates following chemotherapy and radiation therapy range from 15% to 21%, although this is expected to be lower following en bloc resection.
- Death results from widespread hematogenous spread.

## Helpful Hints

- En bloc spondylectomy within the axial spine can be very challenging.

## Suggested Readings

Grubb MR, Currier BL, Pritchard DJ, Ebersold MJ. Primary Ewing's sarcoma of the spine. *Spine.* 1994;19(3):309–313.

Marco RA, Gentry JB, Rhines LD, et al. Ewing's sarcoma of the mobile spine. *Spine.* 2005;30(7):769–773.

# Failed Back Surgery Syndrome

## Description

Failed back surgery syndrome describes continued pain following one or more spinal surgeries. The term is controversial as some believe it is not a diagnosis.

## Etiology/Types

- Multiple spine surgeries

## Epidemiology

- Approximately 2,000 cases of failed back surgery syndrome are produced yearly in the United Kingdom.
- Typically involves younger patients.

## Pathogenesis

- Variable

## Risk Factors

- Anxiety
- Depression
- Inability to achieve surgical goal and continued progressive disease
- Inappropriate surgical procedure
- Incorrect diagnosis
- Litigation
- Number of previous surgeries
- Poor patient selection
- Poor surgical technique
- Worker's compensation payments

## Clinical Features

- Pain following surgery suggests the disc may not have been adequately decompressed or the wrong level was chosen
- 1 to 6 months of pain-free status suggests the development of arachnoiditis or infection.
- Greater than 6 months of pain-free status suggests a recurrent disc herniation.
- Leg and back pain suggests arachnoiditis or spinal stenosis.
- Spinal stenosis and scar tissue can coexist.
- Arachnoiditis usually is suspected with more than one lumbar spine surgery.

## Natural History

- Progressive pain and in some cases disability



## Diagnosis

### Differential diagnosis

- Adjacent level disease
- Arachnoiditis
- Discitis
- Inadequate decompression due to a sequestered free fragment, lateral disc herniation, or lateral recess stenosis
- Inadequate fusion
- Recurrent disc herniation
- Spinal instability

### History

- Need to inquire about the number and outcomes of previous surgeries
- Differentiate structural problem versus a medical problem
- Screen for the possibility of addiction disorders, somatization, and depression

### Exam

- Exam may be limited by severe pain.
- Poor outcomes are predicted if patients have more than two out of five nonorganic findings as described by Waddell:
  - Tenderness in a superficial and nonanatomic distribution
  - Simulated axial loading or rotation
  - Distracted straight leg raise
  - Regional weakness or sensory disturbance
  - Overreaction

### Testing

- Laboratory tests include erythrocyte sedimentation rate and blood cultures in suspected disciitis.
- Weight-bearing lateral flexion and extension films are used to rule out instability.
- Pseudoarthosis is suggested if there is lucency around the pedicle screws or if there is a hardware failure.
- MRI with contrast is useful in differentiating between scar tissue and a recurrent disc herniation or disciitis.
- CT myelography is useful for documenting the bony involvement in lateral recess stenosis or central spinal stenosis.
- Electrodiagnostic studies can be used to assess for peripheral neuropathy or nerve injury.
- Selective nerve root blocks can be used to localize the level of the nerve root abnormality.

- Discography can be used to identify a discogenic pain generator following posterior fusion.

### *Pitfalls*

- Inability to identify underlying diagnosis following extensive assessment

## Red Flags

- Progressive neurologic dysfunction
- Bowel or bladder changes

## Treatment

### *Medical*

- Intensive multidisciplinary approach
- NSAIDs
- Muscle relaxants
- Analgesics

### *Exercises*

- General strengthening and stretching has been found to improve function and decrease use of pain medication.

### *Modalities*

- Heat, cold, ultrasound, and transcutaneous electrical nerve stimulation have been used for symptomatic relief of pain and muscle spasms.

### *Injection*

- Trigger point injections for symptoms of myofascial pain
- Zygapophyseal (facet) joint injection
- Medial branch blocks/radiofrequency neurotomy
- Epidural steroid injection for radicular symptoms
- Discography
- Spinal cord stimulation
- Intrathecal pain medication

### *Surgical*

- Revision surgery
- Scar tissue due to arachnoiditis or epidural fibrosis does not respond to repeat surgery.

### *Consults*

- Physical medicine and rehabilitation
- Neurologic or orthopedic-spine surgery
- Pain management
- Psychiatry or psychology

### *Complications of treatment*

- Vascular injury or compartment syndrome
- Initial hardware placement may stretch the nerve roots resulting in pain, which resolves over several weeks to months.
- Hardware failure
- Pain may also worsen following the completion of rehabilitation and returning to work

## Prognosis

- 15% of surgical patients will develop disability and discomfort.
- Postoperative spondylolisthesis ranges from 10% to 12%.
- 5% to 15% of patients develop a recurrent disc herniation.
- One review reported success rates of >50% after the first surgery, 30% after the second surgery, 15% after the third surgery, and 5% after the fourth surgery.
- Up to 36% of patients develop adjacent level disease.

## Helpful Hints

- Caution should be used in discouraging or detracting patients from appropriate diagnosis and treatment regardless of the poor outcomes with multiple spine surgeries.

## Suggested Reading

Hazard RG. Failed back surgery syndrome: surgical and nonsurgical approaches. *Clin Orthop Relat Res.* 2006;443:228–232.

# Fractures, Lower Cervical Spine

## Description

Fractures of the lower cervical spine

## Etiology/Types

- The Allen Ferguson scale is the most common classification system for subaxial cervical spinal injuries.
  - The scale is based on the mechanism of injury, which allows for prediction of bony and ligamentous injury.
  - It is categorized into six fracture types: compression–flexion, vertical compression, distraction flexion, compression extension, distraction extension, and lateral flexion.

## Epidemiology

- Compression–flexion, distraction extension, and lateral flexion injuries each comprise about 20% of subaxial spine fractures.
- Vertical compression injuries make up 15%.
- Distraction flexion injuries make up 10%.

## Pathogenesis

- Compression–flexion injuries are due to increased anterior column compression and posterior column distraction.
  - Subdivided from stage I representing a round and blunted anteriosuperior part of the vertebral body to stage V, >3 mm of retrolisthesis into the central canal, three-column spinal injury
- Vertical compression injuries
  - Subdivided from stage I, central cupping fracture of the endplate, to stage III, posterior displacement of the vertebral body into the central canal
- Distractive flexion injuries
  - Subdivided from stage I, blunting of the anteriosuperior vertebral body with <25% anterior zygapophyseal (facet) joint subluxation, to stage IV, 100% anterolisthesis with canal impingement
- Compression extension injuries
  - Subdivided from stage I, unilateral vertebral arch injuries, to stage V, 100% anterior displacement of the vertebral body
- Distraction extension injuries
  - Subdivided from stage I, anterior longitudinal ligament failure or a transverse fracture through the vertebral body, to stage II, failure of the anterior and posterior longitudinal ligaments
- Lateral flexion injuries
  - Subdivided from stage I, ipsilateral fractures of the vertebral body and vertebral arch, to stage II, fracture with displacement of the ipsilateral arch fracture or contralateral ligamentous failure

## Risk Factors

- Motor vehicle accidents
- Trauma, including falls or sports-related injuries

## Clinical Features

- Compression–flexion injuries most often affect C4, C5, and C6 levels and are associated with motor vehicle and diving accidents.
- Vertical compression injuries most commonly affect C6 and C7 levels and are associated with blunt trauma or a direct blow to the head due to a motor vehicle accident or diving accident.
- Compression–extension injuries are often posterior element fractures resulting from motor vehicle accidents or diving accidents.
- Distraction extension injuries are most commonly due to motor vehicle accidents or falls.
- Lateral flexion injuries are commonly a result of a motor vehicle accident or sports-related injury.

## Natural History

- Onset with acute injuries/trauma

## Diagnosis

### *Differential diagnosis*

- None

### *History*

- History of an acute injury/trauma
- Neck pain

### *Exam*

- Decreased neck range of motion
- Bony tenderness
- Soft tissue swelling
- Neurologic dysfunction
- Spinal cord injury

### *Testing*

- X-rays, MRI, and CT to assess the extent of cervical spine injury

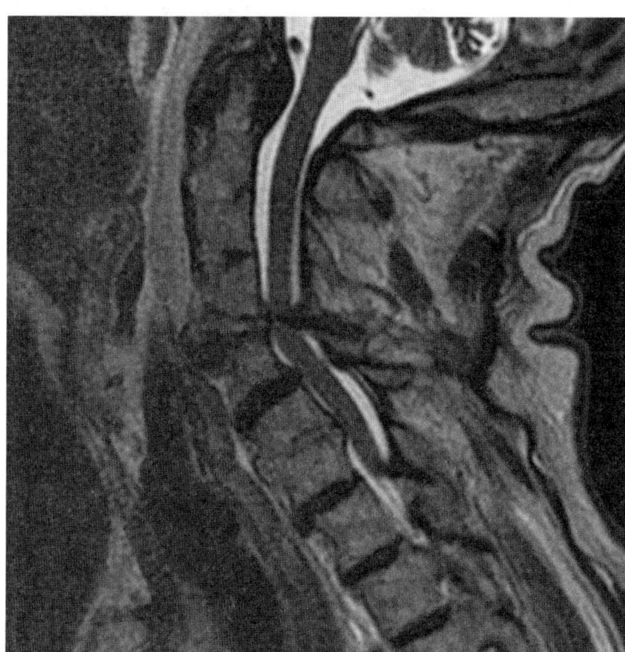

Sagittal cervical T2-weighted magnetic resonance image demonstrating a stage III vertical compression injury of the C4 vertebral body with central canal compromise. (Courtesy of Keith Hentel, MD.)

### *Pitfalls*

- Unstable spine

## Red Flags

- Progressive neurologic deficits
- Radiographic or physical evidence of an unstable spine

## Treatment

### *Medical*

- Immediate evaluation
- Cervical orthosis

### *Exercises*

- None

### *Modalities*

- None

### *Injection*

- None

### *Surgical*

- Halo-vest immobilization
- Decompression and fusion

### *Consults*

- Neurologic or orthopedic-spine surgery
- Physical medicine and rehabilitation for postsurgical rehabilitation

### *Complications of treatment*

- Surgical complications including bleeding, infection, and neurologic injury

## Prognosis

- Compression–flexion injuries increase the risk of complete spinal cord injury from 38% for stage III to 91% for stage V.

## Helpful Hints

- Fully screen for a cervical fracture following acute injury

## Suggested Reading

Klein GR, Vaccaro AR. Cervical spine trauma: upper and lower. In: Vaccaro AR, Betz RR, Zeidman SM, eds. *Principles and Practice of Spine Surgery*. Philadelphia, PA: Mosby; 2003:441–462.

# Fractures, Upper Cervical Spine

## Description
Fractures of the upper cervical spine

## Etiology/Types
- Occipital condyle fractures
- Atlanto-occipital dislocations
- Atlas fractures
- Odontoid fractures
- Traumatic spondylolisthesis of the axis
- Atlantoaxial subluxation

## Epidemiology
- Occipital condyle fractures comprise 16% of cervical spine fractures.
- Atlas fractures and odontoid fractures comprise 13% to 15% of all cervical spine fractures.
- Traumatic spondylolisthesis of the axis comprises 12% to 18% of cervical spine fractures.

## Pathogenesis
- Occipital condyle fractures result from axial compression with a lateral or anterior shear force with or without a rotatory component, types I to III
- Atlanto-occipital dislocations are related to longitudinal traction with a concomitant hyperextension force, types I to III.
- Atlas fractures are related to an axial load with concomitant flexion or extension forces, type I to III.
  - Type III is also known as Jefferson (burst) fracture of the atlas.
- Odontoid fracture is related to hyperflexion or hyperextension forces, types I to III.
- Traumatic spondylolisthesis of the axis
  - Hangman's fracture is due to an axial traction force with hyperextension causing a fracture of the bilateral C2 pars interarticularis and anterolisthesis of C2 on C3, types I to III.
- Atlantoaxial subluxation, types I to IV

## Risk Factors
- Diving/falls
- Head trauma
- Trauma/motor vehicle accidents

## Clinical Features
- Occipital condyle fractures are usually due to a blow to the head.
  - Variable presentation from no neurologic deficit, impaired cranial nerves IX, X, XI, XII to complete tetraplegia
- Atlanto-occipital dislocation presentations are variable with significant neurologic deficits, including brainstem, cranial nerve VII–X, and cervical nerve root injuries.
- Atlas fractures are commonly a result of motor vehicle accidents, direct falls, diving, or blows to the head; associated with other cervical injuries.
  - Upper neck and suboccipital pain; headaches related to trauma; neurologic injuries are rare; may affect cranial nerves IX, X, XI, and XII
- Odontoid fractures result in neurologic abnormalities in up to 25% cases.
- Traumatic spondylolisthesis of the axis is most commonly due to motor vehicle accidents.
  - Neck pain
  - Neurologic dysfunction is rare due to the large central canal diameter.
- Atlantoaxial subluxation results in decreased neck range of motion and suboccipital pain.

## Natural History
- Onset with acute injuries

## Diagnosis

### Differential diagnosis
- None

### History
- History of an acute injury
- Neck pain
- Neurologic symptoms

### Exam
- Decreased neck range of motion
- Bony tenderness
- Soft tissue swelling
- Neurologic dysfunction
- Spinal cord injury

### Testing
- Occipital condyle fractures or suspected C1 fractures are best imaged with CT.
- Lateral masses are measured using an odontoid X-ray view or axial CT views.
- MRI is useful to assess soft tissue and ligamentous injury.

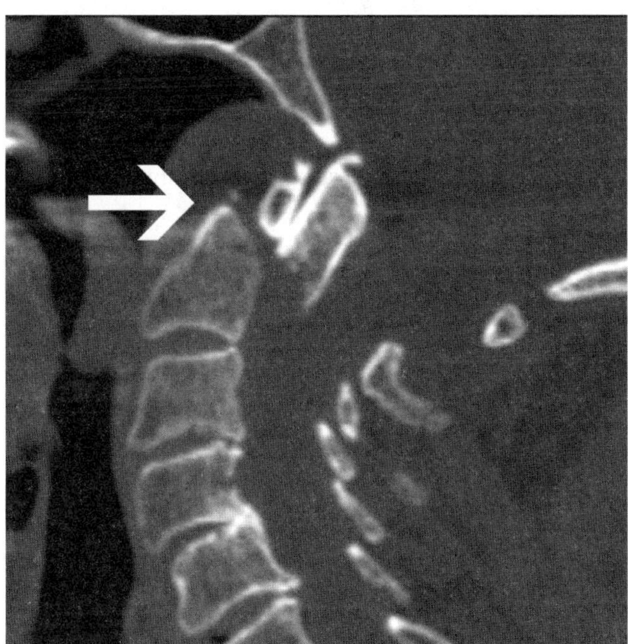

Sagittal cervical reformatted computed tomography scan demonstrating an odontoid (C2) fracture. (Courtesy of Keith Hentel, MD.)

### *Pitfalls*

- Missed fractures

## Red Flags

- Progressive neurologic deficits/spinal cord injury
- Unstable spine

## Treatment

### *Medical*

- Occipital condylar fractures may be treated with a hard cervical collar for 2 to 3 months.
- Atlas fractures that are isolated and stable may be treated with a hard cervical collar.
- Odontoid fractures without ligamentous injury can be treated in a cervical orthosis for 3 months.
- Isolated Jefferson fractures have been successfully treated using a hard cervical collar for 12 weeks.

### *Exercises*

- None

### *Modalities*

- None

### *Injection*

- None

### *Surgical*

- Occipital condylar fractures, atlas fractures, or hangman's fractures: halo-vest immobilization or surgical stabilization
- Atlanto-occipital dislocations, odontoid fractures, atlantoaxial subluxation: halo-vest immobilization and eventual surgical stabilization

### *Consults*

- Neurologic or orthopedic-spine surgery
- Physical medicine and rehabilitation for postsurgical rehabilitation

### *Complications of treatment*

- Complications include bleeding, infection, neurologic injury, or death.

## Prognosis

- Atlanto-occipital dislocations are associated with a high mortality.
- Odontoid fractures are associated with a 10% mortality rate.
- Hangman's fractures have a mortality rate of up to 40%.

## Helpful Hints

- Fully screen for a cervical fracture

## Suggested Reading

Klein GR, Vaccaro AR. Cervical spine trauma: upper and lower. In: Vaccaro AR, Betz RR, Zeidman SM, eds. *Principles and Practice of Spine Surgery*. Philadelphia, PA: Mosby; 2003:441–462.

# Fractures, Sacrum

## Description

Fractures of the sacrum

## Etiology/Types

- Fracture related to acute injury
- Sacral insufficiency fracture

## Epidemiology

- About 1% of older patients presenting with low back pain have a sacral insufficiency fracture.

## Pathogenesis

- The sacrum is classified into three fracture zones:
  - Zone 1, the ala region (lateral ala fracture), is occasionally associated with the fifth lumbar root injury.
  - Zone 2, sacral foramina region (fracture line through one or more sacral foramen and may include the lateral ala), is associated with sciatica and occasionally bladder dysfunction.
  - Zone 3, the central sacral canal (can also include zone 1 and 2 fractures as well), is associated with saddle anesthesia and loss of sphincter control.
- Pelvic ring fractures are associated with transverse type fractures at the S2 and S3 levels (zone 3).

## Risk Factors

- Amenorrheic female long distance runners
- Corticosteroid use
- Falls
- High-energy injuries/motor vehicle accidents
- Multiple myeloma
- Obesity
- Osteopenia or osteoporosis
- Radiation
- Rheumatoid arthritis

## Clinical Features

- Zone 1 fractures are commonly associated with lateral compression pelvic injuries, such as those sustained in a car-versus-pedestrian accident.
- Zone 3 fractures are associated with burst fractures or fracture dislocations associated with high-energy impact.
- 25% of sacral fractures result in neurologic injury; 5.9% in zone 1, 28.4% in zone 2, and 56.7% in zone 3.
- 80% to 90% of pelvic fractures have an associated sacral fracture.
- Neurologic findings are rare with sacral insufficiency fractures.

## Natural History

- Onset with or without acute injury

## Diagnosis

### *Differential diagnosis*

- None

### *History*

- Mechanism of injury
- Neurologic symptoms associated with the injury

### *Exam*

- Ankle dorsiflexion/plantar flexion, hip extension, knee flexion weakness
- Sensory loss in the sacral distribution
- S2–S5 injury manifests as bowel and bladder incontinence as well as sexual dysfunction.
- Diminished ankle jerk with S1 root lesions
- Dull lower back pain that is worsened with direct palpation over the sacrum

### *Testing*

- CT is used to evaluate complex sacral fractures or fractures associated with neurologic deficits.

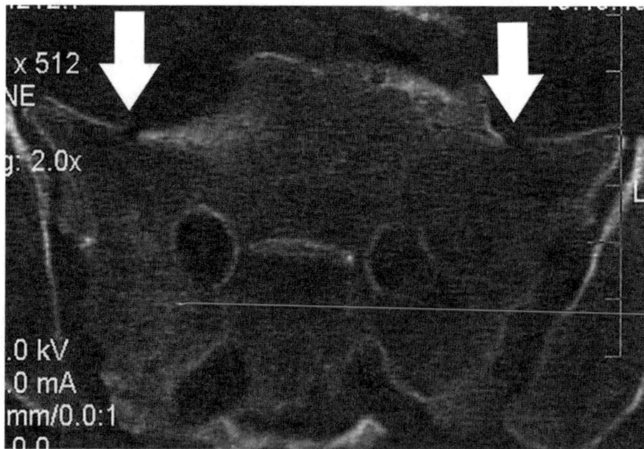


Coronal sacral reformatted computed tomography scan demonstrating a zone 1 lateral ala fracture (arrows). (Adapted from Fast A, Goldsher D. *Navigating the Adult Spine: Bridging Clinical Practice and Neuroradiology.* New York: Demos Medical Publishing, 2007:99.)

- Transverse fractures may be seen on sagittal CT reconstructions
- MRI demonstrates bony edema associated with a fracture.
- Electrodiagnostic studies can localize the area of injury and provide a prognosis for nerve recovery
- Bone scans note a longitudinal fracture line, parallel to the sacroiliac joint

### *Pitfalls*

- Positive bone scans can often be mistaken for metastatic disease.
- Zone 1 ala region fractures can be associated with L5 root injury.

## Red Flags

- Neurologic deficits
- Unstable pelvic ring

## Treatment

### *Medical*

- Neurologically stable fractures in zones 1 and 2 can be managed with bed rest followed by progressive mobilization.
- Closed reduction can be done on vertically displaced alar fractures with L5 root impingement with bed rest, skeletal traction, and or a hip spica cast.
- Transverse fractures above S1–S2 can be treated with bed rest and traction.
- Sacral insufficiency fractures often improve within 3 to 5 weeks, although they may take up to 12 months with bed rest and analgesics.

### *Exercises*

- Focus on body mechanics training, transfer training, extensor strengthening

### *Modalities*

- Have been used for symptomatic relief following the acute period

### *Injection*

- Sacroplasty

### *Surgical*

- Posterior laminectomy and decompression of the sacral neural structures can provide the best chance of recovery.
- Displaced zone 2 fractures should be realigned surgically.

### *Consults*

- Neurologic or orthopedic-spine surgery
- Physical medicine and rehabilitation

### *Complications of treatment*

- Severe long-term pain and mobility deficits are related to lumbosacral plexus injury with pelvic trauma.

## Prognosis

- Sacral stress fractures usually take about 2 months before patients are allowed to return to normal activity.
- Long-term gait dysfunction related to lumbosacral plexus injury with pelvic trauma is best predicted with absent peroneal conduction to the extensor digitorum brevis muscle and absent motor units in the anterior tibialis muscle.

## Helpful Hints

- Functional predictions cannot be made based on fracture characteristics.

## Suggested Reading

Denis F, Davis S, Comfort T. Sacral fractures: an important problem. Retrospective analysis of 236 cases. *Clin Orthop Relat Res.* 1988;227:67–81.

# Fractures, Thoracolumbar Spine

## Description

Fractures of the thoracolumbar spine

## Etiology/Types

- Burst fracture
- Compression fracture
- Fracture dislocations
- Flexion distraction injuries

## Epidemiology

- 15,000 major thoracolumbar injuries per year
- 5,000 result in significant neurologic complications
- 60% of all thoracolumbar injuries occur between T11 and L1.
- Burst fracture is most common.
- Male predominance
- Falls are more common in the elderly population.

## Pathogenesis

- T2–T10 levels resist flexion and extension.
- Central canal of the thoracic spine is narrow, increasing the risk of spinal cord injury.
- T11–L1 is the thoracolumbar junction (transition zone), where most injuries occur.
- Burst fractures are the most common injury.
- Retropulsed bone is usually resorbed and spinal stability is often reestablished with a healed fracture.

## Risk Factors

- Falls
- Flexion distraction injuries—seat belt injuries
- Fracture dislocations—high-energy injuries
- Motor vehicle accidents/trauma

## Clinical Features

- Spine deformity
- Neurologic dysfunction
- Spinal cord injury

## Natural History

- Onset with acute injuries

## Diagnosis

### *Differential diagnosis*

- Osteoporotic-compression fracture
- Neoplasm



### *History*

- Mechanism of injury
- Neurologic symptoms associated with the injury

### *Exam*

- Assess for spine deformity
- Palpate for tender regions and gaps between the spinous processes
- Assess over serial examinations, taking care to note any progressive neurologic deficits
- Assess for spinal shock, which manifests as an absence of motor, sensory, or deep tendon reflexes below the level of injury
- Spinal cord injury assessment

### *Testing*

- X-rays are used to screen all patients for injuries to the spine.
- MRI is used to assess the posterior ligamentous region, as well as the central canal and the status of the spinal cord.
- CT is used to assess the middle spinal column and posterior zygapophyseal (facet) joints.

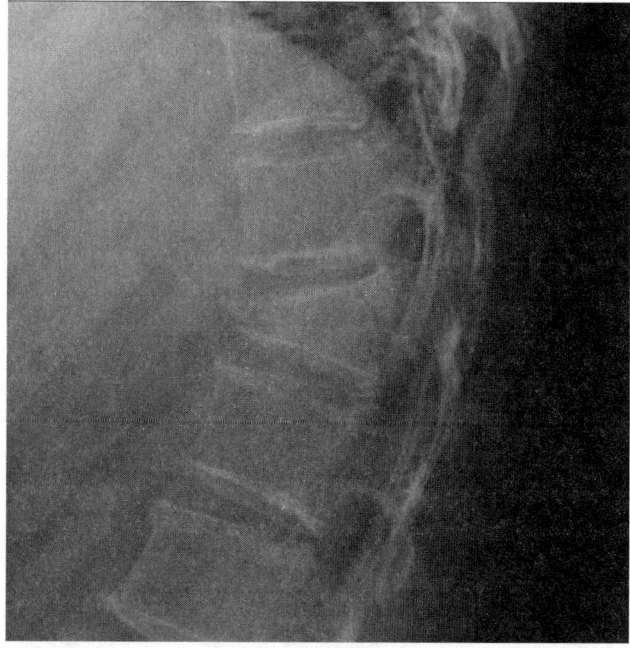

Lateral lumbar plain radiograph demonstrating a T12 compression fracture primarily involving the anterior column.

*Pitfalls*

- Missed fractures
- Overlooked spinal cord injury

## Red Flags

- Progressive neurologic deficits
- Unstable spine

## Treatment

*Medical*

- Stable thoracolumbar fractures can be treated nonsurgically with early ambulation.
- Stable burst fractures with no neurologic deficits may be treated with a hyperextension brace or custom orthosis
- Upper thoracic–compression fractures are stabilized by the rib cage and often do not need bracing.
- Compression fractures that involve the anterior column are stable.
- Thoracolumbar and lumbar fractures can be braced with an extension brace or a thoracolumbosacral orthosis.

*Exercises*

- Focus on body mechanics training, transfer training, and extensor strengthening

*Modalities*

- Have been used for symptomatic relief following the acute period

*Injection*

- Trigger point injections have been used for symptomatic relief following the acute period.

*Surgical*

- Surgical fusion for complete dislocations, significant ligamentous, or soft tissue disruption, compression fractures that involve the posterior ligamentous column, and deterioration with nonoperative care.
- Burst fractures are treated surgically if there are neurologic deficits, vertebral body height loss of >50%, angulation >20 degrees, lateral tilt >10 degrees, canal compromise >50 degrees, or posterior ligament disruption
- Flexion distraction injuries are treated surgically if there is ligamentous disruption.

*Consults*

- Neurologic or orthopedic-spine surgery
- Physical medicine and rehabilitation

*Complications of treatment*

- The most common cause of mortality is thromboembolism especially in complete spinal cord injury.
- Surgical complications including bleeding, infection, and neurologic injury

## Prognosis

- At 2-year follow-up of thoracolumbar burst fractures, 49% had excellent pain and functional outcomes, 90% had satisfactory work status.
- 20-year follow-up of burst fractures without neurologic compromise, 88% of patients were able to work at their usual level of activity.

## Helpful Hints

- Isolated L5 transverse process fracture is often associated with an underlying pelvic or sacral fracture.

## Suggested Reading

Wood K, Buttermann G, Mehbod A, Garvey T, Jhanjee R, Sechriest V. Operative compared with nonoperative treatment of a thoracolumbar burst fracture without neurological deficit. A prospective, randomized study. *J Bone Joint Surg Am.* 2003;85-A(5):773–781.

# Giant Cell Tumor

## Description

A giant cell tumor develops from non–bone-forming connective tissue and is the most common locally aggressive tumor with malignant potential.

## Etiology/Types

- Originate from the non–bone-forming connective tissue within the bone marrow
- Begins growing once skeletal maturity has occurred

## Epidemiology

- Comprise 21% of all benign bone tumors and 5% of primary bone tumors
- Less than 10% become malignant
- Average age at diagnosis is 20 to 40 years
- Described in patients from 2 to 66 years of age
- Males are more likely to be diagnosed with a malignant tumor.
- Females are more likely to be diagnosed with a benign tumor.

## Pathogenesis

- Unknown

## Risk Factors

- Unknown

## Clinical Features

- Most commonly found at the ends of long bones, such as the knee
- 8% to 12% of cases involve the axial spine
- In the axial spine, 68% occur in the sacrum, 11% occur in the cervical and lumbar spine, and 10% occur in the thoracic spine.
- Microscopically, contains a large number of osteoblast-like giant cells separated by mononuclear stromal cells.
- 88% of patients have neurologic dysfunction, which includes leg weakness or paresthesias, including perineal hypoesthesias, bowel and bladder dysfunction or paraplegia.
- Cervical spinal involvement includes dysphagia.

## Natural History

- Progressive enlargement



## Diagnosis

### *Differential diagnosis*

- Aneurysmal bone cyst
- Brown tumor of hyperparathyroidism
- Chondroblastoma
- Chondromyxoid fibroma
- Enchondroma
- Fibrous dysplasia
- Simple bone cyst
- Ossifying or nonossifying fibroma
- Osteoblastoma
- Osteosarcoma

### *History*

- Intermittent aching pain in the sacrum, lumbar, or cervical spine

### *Exam*

- Axial spine or sacral tenderness
- Localized swelling may be evident with superficial presentation.
- Kyphosis and muscle spasm may also be noted in the cervical or lumbar region at the site of involvement.
- Extracolonic mass on rectal examination with sacral presentations
- Neurologic dysfunction

### *Testing*

- Laboratory tests may demonstrate anemia and an elevated erythrocyte sedimentation rate.
  - Serum calcium, phosphorus, and alkaline phosphatase tests can be used to differentiate the tumor from malignant giant cell tumor, hyperparathyroidism, and Paget's disease.
- X-rays may demonstrate an osteolytic lesion without surrounding reactive sclerosis or matrix mineralization.
- CT can be used to define the extent of bony destruction.
- MRI notes a low to intermediate signal on T1-weighted images and often low to high signal intensity on T2-weighted images.
  - Can be used to evaluate the extraosseous spread
  - Contrast enhancement varies

### *Pitfalls*

- Delay in diagnosis up to 3 years
- Sacral presentations may be missed on routine X-rays.

## Red Flags

- Neurologic deficits
- Unstable spine

## Treatment

### Medical

- Staging is done with CT to determine bony involvement, MRI to assess the extraosseous spread

### Exercises

- None

### Modalities

- None

### Injection

- None

### Surgical

- En bloc excision is the treatment of choice.
- Radical excision is the treatment of choice followed by radiation, but surgery is often difficult or impossible.
- Curettage has been shown to have a 50% recurrence rate in 5 years.
- Embolization has been considered for presurgical treatment to decrease risk of profound bleeding or to eliminate the need for radiation.

### Consults

- Neurologic or orthopedic-spine surgery
- Radiation oncology

### Complications of treatment

- Can be difficult to treat due to unpredictable behavior and location
- Radiation of giant cell tumors of the extremities is contraindicated due to the risk of malignant transformation
- The condition has been misdiagnosed as a radiculpathy or lumbar disc herniation and some even undergo discectomy.

## Prognosis

- Prognosis is based on complete tumor removal.
- Up to 50% of benign giant cell tumors recur.
- Complete or partial en bloc resection of the sacrum often includes the sacrifice of sacral nerve roots resulting in the loss of bowel, bladder, and sexual function.
- Mortality is associated with local invasion, malignant transformation, or renal failure due to neurogenic bladder.
- Mortality is 33% at 4 years following an extensive resection and reconstruction of a vertebral or sacral lesion.

## Helpful Hints

- 44% recurrence rate for all giant cell tumors, with a 16.5% to 28% recurrence rate in the spine
- Neurologic deficits may be irreversible if there is a delay of more than 3 months before decompression

## Suggested Readings

Dahlin DC. Giant-cell tumor of vertebrae above the sacrum: a review of 31 cases. *Cancer.* 1977;39(3):1350–1356.

Turcotte RE, Sim FH, Unni KK. Giant cell tumor of the sacrum. *Clin Orthop Relat Res.* 1993;(291):215–221.

# Hemangiomas

## Description

Hemangiomas are benign vascular lesions in soft tissues or bones that are made up of cavernous, capillary, or venous blood vessels.

## Etiology/Types

- Unknown

## Epidemiology

- Less than 1% of symptomatic primary bone tumors
- Prevalence increases with age and is most often identified by the fourth or fifth decade.
- Found in up to 12% of autopsies
- No gender preference

## Pathogenesis

- Unknown

## Risk Factors

- Increased intra-abdominal venous pressure during the third trimester of pregnancy may cause increased paravertebral venous plexus flow, causing a previously asymptomatic hemangioma to expand and bleed, resulting in associated neurologic deficits.

## Clinical Features

- Approximately 50% are found in the thoracic spine, followed by 39% in the lumbar spine and 7% in the cervical spine.
- Neurologic symptoms develop by enlargement of the vertebral body, leading to distortion or narrowing of the central canal, tumor extension into the epidural space, or compression fracture and associated bleeding into the epidural space
- Multiple hemangiomas may cause spinal cord compression.
- Neurologic involvement is most common in the thoracic spine.
- May be related to pregnancy
- Rarely associated with spinal cord compression

## Natural History

- Ranges from no progression over many years to progressive enlargement over months

## Diagnosis

### *Differential diagnosis*

- Angiolipoma
- Gorham's disease
- Metastasis
- Osler-Weber-Rendu disease
- Paget's disease
- Skeletal lymphangiomatosis

### *History*

- Localized back or neck pain
- Tenderness over the involved vertebral body
- Associated muscle spasm
- Neurologic dysfunction related to cord compression

### *Exam*

- Palpable swelling may be noted
- Tenderness to palpation of the involved vertebral body
- Associated muscle spasm
- Kyphosis related to a thoracic compression fracture
- Neurologic dysfunction

### *Testing*

- X-rays demonstrate coarse vertical vertebral striations or a corduroy appearance of the vertebral body,

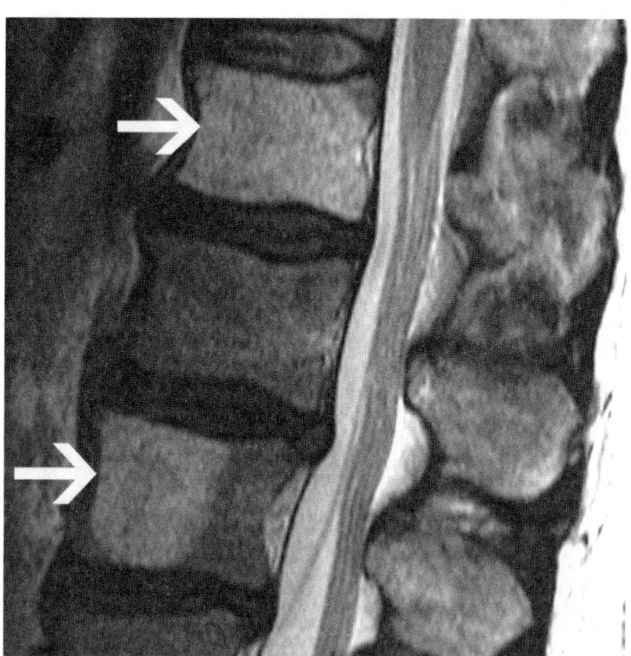

Sagittal lumbar T2-weighted magnetic resonance image demonstrating increased signal within the vertebral bodies (arrows), compatible with a hemangioma. (Adapted from Fast A, Goldsher D. *Navigating the Adult Spine: Bridging Clinical Practice and Neuroradiology.* New York: Demos Medical Publishing, 2007:112.)

described as a "honeycomb" appearance; the vertebral body may be enlarged.

- Asymptomatic hemangiomas commonly appear on MRI in a portion of the lumbar vertebral body
- The increased T1 signal corresponds to the fatty stroma (relative proportion of adipocytes) and the increased T2 signal corresponds to the vasculature (vessels and interstitial edema).
- CT can demonstrate bony extension and possible involvement of the pedicle or neural arch.
- Bone scan demonstrates increased uptake at the site of the hemangioma.

### *Pitfalls*

- In 10% of cases with neurologic manifestations, pregnancy is a precipitating factor.

## Red Flags

- Progressive neurologic deficits
- Unstable spine

## Treatment

### *Medical*

- Symptoms may improve with unchanged radiographic appearance.
- Hemangiomas respond to radiation treatment.

### *Exercises*

- None

### *Modalities*

- None

### *Injection*

- Percutaneous vertebral augmentation can be used to strengthen the vertebral body if there is a risk of vertebral collapse and can provide symptomatic pain relief.

### *Surgical*

- Spinal cord compression requires surgical decompression with or without postoperative radiation.
- Laminectomy can be associated with significant morbidity and mortality due to the potential of significant hemorrhage.
- Angiography can be used for preoperative embolization to decrease the risk of hemorrhage.
- Acute spinal cord injury requires surgical decompression.
- Spinal instability may require fusion.

### *Consults*

- Neurologic or orthopedic-spine surgery

### *Complications of treatment*

- Hemorrhage with laminectomy
- Delayed radiation-induced sarcoma

## Prognosis

- A 6-year follow-up of asymptomatic patients demonstrated no interval radiographic change of intraosseous lesions.
- A 9-year follow-up of patients describing localized pain thought to be related to the vertebral hemangioma did not have neurologic changes or imaging changes

## Helpful Hints

- Management includes careful observation.

## Suggested Readings

Acosta FL Jr, Sanai N, Chi JH, et al. Comprehensive management of symptomatic and aggressive vertebral hemangiomas. *Neurosurg Clin N Am*. 2008;19(1):17–29.

Fox MW, Onofrio BM. The natural history and management of symptomatic and asymptomatic vertebral hemangiomas. *J Neurosurg*. 1993;78(1):36–45.

# Hemoglobinopathies (Sickle Cell Disease, Thalassemia)

## Description

Hemoglobinopathies describe a series of disorders that cause a defect in the production of hemoglobin.

## Etiology/Types

- Sickle cell anemia—hemoglobin SS
- β-thalassemia includes thalassemia major, intermedia trait, and a silent carrier.
- Other less common variants exist.

## Epidemiology

- Sickle cell anemia is found in 1 of 625 Americans of African descent.

## Pathogenesis

- Adult hemoglobin (hemoglobin A) consists of two pairs of coiled α and β chains.
- Hemoglobin S decreases solubility with deoxygenation, causing it to take on an irreversible "sickle" shape.
- Bone marrow hyperplasia and chronic anemia
- Thalassemia results from abnormal production of the α chain and its β, γ, or δ chains, which causes early erythrocyte destruction.
- Tissue deoxygenation leads to bone marrow hyperplasia in the axial spine, increasing the risk of fractures.

## Risk Factors

- African, Asian, or Mediterranean descent
- Dehydration, infection, fever, or acidosis

## Clinical Features

- Sickle cell disease
  - Acute low back with radiation and extremity pain are the most common complaint lasting about 4 to 5 days with no residual effects.
  - Abdominal pain
  - Bone infarction
  - Joint effusion or hemarthrosis
  - Septic arthritis
  - Osteomyelitis
  - Vertebral body compression fractures
  - Increased thoracic kyphosis and lumbar lordosis
- Thalassemia results in organomegaly, osteopenia, spinal cord compression due to extramedullary hematopoesis.

## Natural History

- Variable

## Diagnosis

### *Differential diagnosis*

- Abdominal disorders
- Other causes of anemia

### *History*

- Acute low back pain with radiation and extremity pain
- Abdominal pain
- Muscle spasm

### *Exam*

- Febrile
- Distress in acute sickling crises
- Tenderness in the affected areas
- Abdominal tenderness with normal bowel sounds
- Thalassemia patients have altered skin pigmentation and hepatosplenomegaly.
- Marrow hyperplasia in thalassemia patients causes bony expansion, resulting in frontal bossing and maxillary prominence.

### *Testing*

- Laboratory studies demonstrate anemia, leukocytosis, and mild thrombocytopenia with sickled cells and Howell-Jolly bodies.
- Thalassemia results in a hypochromic, microcytic blood smear.
- X-rays demonstrate cortical thinning and loss of bony trabeculae due to marrow hyperplasia.
- Skull X-ray demonstrates a "hair-on-end" appearance.
- Bone scan demonstrates increased uptake in areas of increased bone marrow.
- MRI demonstrates replacement of fat by marrow.

### *Pitfalls*

- Differentiating bone infarction from osteomyelitis

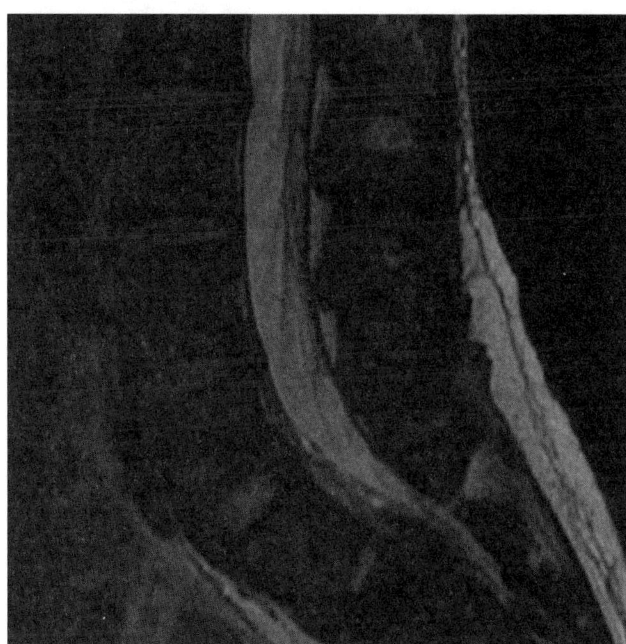

Sagittal lumbar T2-weighted magnetic resonance image demonstrating decreased signal throughout the vertebral bodies due to replacement of normal fatty stroma by hematopoietic cells in β-thalassemia.

## Red Flags

- Joint effusion or hemarthrosis
- Septic arthritis/osteomyelitis
- Pneumonia/pulmonary infarction
- Vertebral body compression fractures

## Treatment

### *Medical*

- Hydration
- Analgesics, opioids
- Hydroxyurea to increase fetal hemoglobin
- Sulphasalazine
- In thalassemia, blood transfusions suppress marrow hyperplasia resulting in bony pathology. Iron chelation is used to decrease iron overload; radiation to stop the overgrowth of extramedullary marrow.
- Bone marrow transplantation
- Lumbar bracing for vertebral body fractures or collapse

### *Exercises*

- Sickle cell patients should exercise with caution due to an increased risk of acute sickle crisis.
- Thalassemia patients have a diminished exercise capacity.

### *Modalities*

- Contraindicated in an acute crisis

### *Injection*

- None

### *Surgical*

- Surgical decompression of extramedullary marrow tissue compressing the spinal cord in thalassemia patients, followed by radiation treatment

### *Consults*

- Hematology
- Neurological or orthopedic-spine surgery

### *Complications of treatment*

- Multiple blood transfusions in thalassemia patients increase the risk of infectious disease, iron overload, and formation of antibodies.
- Surgical risk due to low platelet count, poor bone mass, anemia, or cardiomyopathy

## Prognosis

- Sickle cell patients and thalassemia patients may live up to the fourth decade.

## Helpful Hints

- Patients may appear comfortable but report excruciating pain.

## Suggested Reading

Cordner S, De Ceulaer K. Musculoskeletal manifestations of hemoglobinopathies. *Curr Opin Rheumatol.* 2003;15(1):44–47.

# Hyperparathyroidism

## Description

Hyperparathyroidism causes the increased secretion of parathyroid hormone (PTH) resulting in bone loss and spinal deformity from fractures of the vertebral body.

## Etiology/Types

- Primary hyperparathyroidism is a result of abnormal growth of the parathyroid glands due to an adenoma, multiple adenomas, carcinoma, or diffuse hyperplasia.
- Secondary hyperparathyroidism is the increased secretion of PTH in response to low serum calcium caused by kidney dysfunction or decreased vitamin D metabolism.

## Epidemiology

- Unknown prevalence
- Male to female ratio is 1:3
- Hyperparathyroidism is associated with multiple endocrine neoplasia type I and IIa syndromes.

## Pathogenesis

- PTH is responsible for maintaining serum calcium levels by synthesizing the active form of vitamin D, stimulating intestinal and renal uptake of calcium, activating osteoclastic bony resorption, and increasing phosphate excretion.
- Persistently elevated PTH causes bony demineralization.

## Risk Factors

- Multiple endocrine neoplasms type I and IIa

## Clinical Features

- Bone pain or vertebral body compression fracture
- 20% report generalized myalgias and arthralgias.
- 10% to 20% of patients also develop nephrolithiasis.
- 25% of patients are at risk for osteopenia and vertebral fractures.
- 50% of patients with slight serum calcium elevations may report weakness and fatigue.
- 20% describe gastrointestinal symptoms such as nausea, vomiting, constipation, anorexia, abdominal pain.
- 3.8% of patients also present with pseudogout.
- Other neurologic changes include changes in mental status and coma.
- Renal failure
- Hypertension

## Natural History

- Vertebral fractures due to progressive kyphosis with associated constitutional symptoms such as abdominal pain, renal failure, hypertension, mental status changes, and coma

## Diagnosis

### *Differential diagnosis*

- Hypophosphatemia
- Neoplasms
- Sarcoidosis

### *History*

- Deep bony pain
- Muscle and joint pain
- Weakness and fatigue
- Nausea and vomiting

### *Exam*

- Vertebral body compression fractures may be noted with tenderness to palpation of the involved bony segment with associated local muscle spasm.

### *Testing*

- 96% of primary hyperparathyroidism patients demonstrate increased serum calcium levels.
- Low serum phosphorus
- Elevated serum alkaline phosphatase and chloride
- Elevated urinary calcium secretion
- Secondary hyperparathyroidism demonstrates elevated serum phosphorus levels and rarely demonstrates increased serum calcium levels.
- PTH assay
- Bone biopsy, which is rarely done, demonstrates increased osteoclasts
- Electrocardiogram may demonstrate a shortened QT interval
- X-rays demonstrate subperiosteal bone resorption on the radial aspects of the middle phalanges, resorption of the terminal tufts of the phalanges, cystic lesions in the long bones, and a "salt and pepper" appearance in the skull.
- Resorption may occur at the pubic symphysis along with sclerosis of the sacroiliac joints, which may result in sacroiliac joint instability.
- Anterior wedging and osteopenia of the vertebral bodies
- Secondary hyperparathyroidism results in arterial calcification and osteosclerosis of soft tissues.

- Bone scan is used to identify affected parathyroid tissue.
- SPECT may be used to detect a parathyroid adenoma.
- Enlarged glands can be identified with CT or ultrasound.

### *Pitfalls*

- Overlooked diagnosis

## Red Flags

- Changes in mental status, coma, muscle weakness, hypotonia, fatigue, anorexia, renal failure, hypertension

## Treatment

### *Medical*

- No effective medical treatment for primary hyperparathyroidism.
- NSAIDs or analgesics for vertebral body compression fractures.

### *Exercises*

- General strengthening and stretching

### *Modalities*

- Heat, cold, ultrasound, and transcutaneous electrical nerve stimulation have been used for symptomatic relief of pain and muscle spasms.

### *Injection*

- Percutaneous vertebral augmentation for treatment of compression fractures

### *Surgical*

- Surgical resection of affected parathyroid tissue is the most definitive treatment.
- Postoperative therapy may include calcium and vitamin D, phosphorus, and magnesium.
- Treatment of secondary hyperparathyroidism requires control of the underlying disease.

### *Consults*

- Endocrinology
- Otolaryngology

### *Complications of treatment*

- Complications related to surgery

## Prognosis

- Patients who are asymptomatic with mildly elevated serum calcium may be followed.
- Patients who become symptomatic require surgical removal and occasionally may require a reoperation.
- Bony lesions heal once the source of excess PTH is removed.
- Large cysts may not heal and may result in pathologic fractures.

## Helpful Hints

- Important to screen for possible underlying etiology

## Suggested Reading

Petti GH Jr. Hyperparathyroidism. *Otolaryngol Clin North Am.* 1990;23(2):339–355.

# Low Back Strain

## Description

A low back strain results from an injury to the dynamic muscle stabilizers or static ligamentous structures of the lower back.

## Etiology/Types

- May be associated with mechanical overload or a prolonged abnormal posture

## Epidemiology

- Represents 60% to 70% of all mechanical low back pain presentations

## Pathogenesis

- May be related to ligamentous or muscular injury from excessive tension or stretching
- Muscle fatigue from overuse
- Muscle spasm caused by muscle overload
- Paraspinal muscle deconditioning due to previous injury

## Risk Factors

- Mechanical overload
- Muscle overuse
- Prolonged abnormal posture

## Clinical Features

- Localized or diffuse nonradiating lower back pain
- Worsened with abnormal or static posture

## Natural History

- Usually a self-limiting condition that may last 6 to 12 weeks

## Diagnosis

### *Differential diagnosis*

- Herniated nucleus pulposus
- Osteoarthritis
- Posterior element or vertebral body fractures
- Scoliosis
- Soft tissue or bony trauma
- Spondyloarthropathies
- Tumors

### *History*

- Dull, aching pain
- Localized or diffuse lower back pain
- Possible radiation into the buttocks but not into the lower extremities
- Pain with flexion and/or extension
- Worsened with activity or static postures and improved with recumbency

### *Exam*

- Normal neurologic examination
- Tenderness to palpation of paraspinal muscles, most often at the L5–S1 region
- Decreased lumbar range of motion
- Supraspinatus ligamentous strains are tender with palpation.

### *Testing*

- X-rays are usually normal.
- MRI or CT studies often do not clarify the diagnosis.
- Asymptomatic congenital findings such as spina bifida occulta, lumbarization of the S1, or sacralization of the L5 occur in about 5% of the population.

### *Pitfalls*

- Lack of correlation of the history to the physical examination

## Red Flags

- Neurologic changes
- Soft tissue or bony abnormalities
- Skin rashes
- Severe pain

## Treatment

### *Medical*

- NSAIDs
- Muscle relaxants
- Opioids if the pain is deemed severe
- Limited use of a lumbar corset
- Acupuncture has been described as helpful for symptomatic relief.

### *Exercises*

- Minimal or no bed rest
- Physical activity within the patient's pain tolerance
- Physical therapy and a home exercise program focused on pain control and regaining mobility

### Modalities
- Heat, cold, ultrasound, and transcutaneous electrical nerve stimulation have been used for symptomatic relief of pain and muscle spasms.

### Injection
- Trigger point injections to block the reflexive spasm, if 2 to 4 weeks have passed without significant improvement

### Surgical
- None

### Consults
- Physical medicine and rehabilitation

### Complications of treatment
- Persistent pain for months or years
- Recurrent episodes of increasing frequency and intensity

## Prognosis
- Up to 90% of cases resolve within 2 months.
- Within 3 to 5 years, there is up to a 60% chance of recurrence.

## Helpful Hints
- Generally thought to be a self-limiting condition
- The physician should reassure the patient that no damage will occur with continued activity.

## Suggested Readings
Deyo RA, Weinstein JN. Low back pain. *N Engl J Med.* 2001;344(5):363–370.

Panagos A, Sable AW, Zuhosky JP, Irwin RW, Sullivan WJ, Foye PM. Industrial medicine and acute musculoskeletal rehabilitation. 1. Diagnostic testing in industrial and acute musculoskeletal injuries. *Arch Phys Med Rehabil.* 2007;88 (3 Suppl 1):S3–S9.

# Lymphoma

## Description

Lymphoma is a malignant disease of lymphoreticular origin that usually arises from the lymph nodes.

## Etiology/Types

- Hodgkin's lymphoma
- Non-Hodgkin's lymphoma
  - B cell lymphoma (most common)
  - T cell lymphoma
  - Natural killer (NK) cell lymphoma
  - Immunodeficiency-associated lymphoproliferative disorders
- Staging (stages I to IV) and grading from low to high for non-Hodgkin's lymphoma allow for further classification
- Unknown etiology

## Epidemiology

- The annual incidence is 40 to 60 cases per million individuals.
- Bony involvement is due to hematogenous spread or direct extension by the tumor.
- Most commonly occurs between 20 and 60 years of age.
- Male to female ratio of 2:1
- The lumbosacral spine is involved in 55% of cases, the thoracic spine 34% of cases, and the cervical spine 11% of cases.

## Pathogenesis

- Generally unknown
- Extraosseous lesions may be related to osteoclastic cytokines produced by the malignant cells.

## Risk Factors

- Autoimmune disease
- Epstein-Barr virus infection
- HIV or HTLV-1 infection
- Increasing age
- Positive family history

## Clinical Features

- Persistent pain over the affected bony region
- Most often invades the axial spine

## Natural History

- Remission is possible in certain types of lymphomas if the disease is not too extensive.
- 5-year survival rate approaches 50%.

## Diagnosis

### *Differential diagnosis*

- Eosinophilic granuloma
- Neoplasm of the breast or prostate
- Paget's disease

### *History*

- Persistent pain over the affected bony area
- Pain is worsened with recumbent position.
- Increased bony pain with the consumption of alcohol
- Multiple lesions may result in constitutional symptoms such as fever.
- Neurologic manifestations with invasion of the peripheral nerves or the central spinal canal

### *Exam*

- Bony tenderness to palpation and a soft tissue mass of the affected bone
- Characteristic tenderness over a pathologic compression fracture
- Neurologic deficits
- Lymphadenopathy and splenomegaly in patients with generalized disease

### *Testing*

- Laboratory studies are usually normal, although anemia with an increased erythrocyte sedimentation rate and increased serum proteins may indicate extension into other tissues.
- Histologic findings include Reed-Steinberg cells, atypical mononuclear cells
- X-rays may demonstrate lytic, sclerotic, periosteal lesions, or a compression fracture
- Primarily invades the vertebral body followed by the posterior elements.
- Bone scan may be used to detect multiple lesions and for monitoring the response to chemotherapy.
- CT is used for staging purposes and to assess bony involvement.
- MRI may detect early changes in bone and lymph node involvement.
- Positron emission tomography (PET) scan
- Bone marrow aspiration

### *Pitfalls*

- Inadequate staging

## Red Flags

- Acute onset of paraparesis or cauda equina syndrome with epidural lymphomas

## Treatment

### Medical

- Radiation therapy and/or chemotherapy based on staging
- Rituximab (anti-CD-20 monoclonal antibodies)
- Stem cell transplant

### Exercises

- None

### Modalities

- None

### Injection

- None

### Surgical

- Surgical decompression is considered in younger patients with rapidly progressive paralysis.

### Consults

- Hematology oncology
- Radiation oncology
- Neurologic or orthopedic-spine surgery

### Complications of treatment

- Complications related to chemotherapeutic agents, surgery, and radiation

## Prognosis

- Significant deficits in mobility may be possible with epidural disease
- The 5-year survival rate is 50%.

## Helpful Hints

- Plain radiographs are an easy tool to use to evaluate for the localized bony manifestations of lymphoma.

## Suggested Readings

Eichler AF, Batchelor TT. Primary central nervous system lymphoma: presentation, diagnosis and staging. *Neurosurg Focus.* 2006;21(5):E15.

Citow JS, Rini B, Wollmann R, Macdonald RL. Isolated, primary extranodal Hodgkin's disease of the spine: case report. *Neurosurgery.* 2001;49(2):453–456.

# Marfan Syndrome

## Description

Marfan syndrome is a connective tissue disorder that primarily affects the skeletal, cardiovascular, and ocular systems.

## Etiology/Types

- Caused by a defect of the fibrillin protein, which is a component of connective tissue microfibrils.

## Epidemiology

- Occurs in 1 in 10,000 individuals.
- 15% of patients are the result of a spontaneous mutation.
- No gender preference

## Pathogenesis

- Autosomal dominant
- Defect of the fibrillin-1 gene on chromosome 15 (*FBN1*)
- Defect in fibrillin synthesis, secretion, and matrix formation

## Risk Factors

- Genetic predisposition

## Clinical Features

- Tall and thin stature
- Long arms compared to the trunk
- Joint laxity
- Loss of thoracic kyphosis
- Multilevel scoliosis occurs in 62% of patients.
- Restrictive lung disease due to scoliosis
- Pectus excavatum (chest depression) and pectus carinatum (pigeon chest) occur in 66% of patients.
- Dural ectasia or a ballooning of the dural sac, may be asymptomatic or result in back pain and headaches
- Atlantoaxial subluxation
- Cervical spinal stenosis
- Arachnodactyly
- 1996 diagnostic criteria include major [4 of 8 skeletal manifestations (see Suggested Readings), lumbosacral dural ectasis, aortic dilatation, and ectopia lentic], and minor criteria (joint hypermobility, myopia, recurrent hernia, mitral valve prolapse).

## Natural History

- Unknown

## Diagnosis

### *Differential diagnosis*

- Ehlers-Danlos syndrome
- Osteogenesis imperfecta

### *History*

- Back pain and headaches may be due to dural ectasia.

### *Exam*

- Tall thin stature
- Neurologic deficits may be due to dural ectasia.
- Pectus excavatum
- Pectus carinatum
- Joint laxity

### *Testing*

- Plain radiographs demonstrate thoracolumbar scoliosis, increased vertebral body height, and posterior scalloping of the vertebral bodies.
- MRI can be useful for assessing possible dural ectasia and cervical spinal stenosis.
- Plain radiographs or CT can be used to assess atlantoaxial subluxation.

### *Pitfalls*

- Dural ectasia

## Red Flags

- Aortic dissection
- Retinal detachment
- Severe mitral valve regurgitation
- Severe pectus excavatum resulting in cardiopulmonary compromise

## Treatment

### *Medical*

- Bracing to prevent progressive scoliosis found to only be successful in 17% of patients.
- Bracing recommended for curves up to 25 degrees and not suggested for curves greater than 40 degrees
- Bracing may begin early in life.

### *Exercises*

- General strengthening
- Stabilization exercises

- Caution with cardiovascular conditioning

### *Modalities*

- Heat, cold, ultrasound, and transcutaneous electrical nerve stimulation have been used for symptomatic relief of pain and muscle spasms.

### *Injection*

- Trigger point injections and epidural steroid injections have been used for symptomatic relief.

### *Surgical*

- Surgical deformity correction is considered with scoliotic curves >40 degrees.

### *Consults*

- Physical medicine and rehabilitation
- Neurologic or orthopedic-spine surgery
- Rheumatology

### *Complications of treatment*

- Variable

## Prognosis

- Continued progressive neurologic decline without treatment
- Average life expectancy is 70 years of age.
- Disease manifestations in the axial spine are unknown

## Helpful Hints

- Be aware of the risk of aortic dissection and dural ectasia that may be the source of axial spine pain.

## Suggested Readings


Demetracopoulos CA, Sponseller PD. Spinal deformities in Marfan syndrome. *Orthop Clin North Am.* 2007;38(4):563–572.

De Paepe A, Devereux RB, Dietz HC, Hennekam RC, Pyeritz RE. Revised diagnostic criteria for the Marfan syndrome. *Am J Med Genet.* 1996;62(4):417–426.

Giampietro PF, Raggio C, Davis JG. Marfan syndrome: orthopedic and genetic review. *Curr Opin Pediatr.* 2002;14(1):35–41.

Sponseller PD, Bhimani M, Solacoff D, Dormans JP. Results of brace treatment of scoliosis in Marfan syndrome. *Spine.* 2000;25(18):2350–2354.

# Meningioma

## Description
Meningioma is a benign tumor that makes up 25% to 45% of all intradural spinal neoplasms.

## Etiology/Types
- Generally unknown, but thought to originate from arachnoidal cells.

## Epidemiology
- Spinal meningiomas make up about 12% of all meningiomas.
- The annual incidence is thought to be 0.5 to 2 per 100,000 individuals.
- Typically affects patients older than 50 years of age
- 80% of patients are female.

## Pathogenesis
- Slow growing tumor
- Remains intradural
- Most common in the thoracic spine with occasional appearance in the cervical and lumbosacral spine

## Risk Factors
- Unknown

## Clinical Features
- The most common complaint is back pain, although other signs include weakness, numbness, parasthesias, and gait ataxia.

## Natural History
- Slow-growing tumor that is first noted with progressive neurologic findings

## Diagnosis

### *Differential diagnosis*
- Abscess
- Chordoma
- Fibroma
- Lipoma
- Lymphoma
- Metastasis
- Vascular malformation

### *History*
- Midline axial or radicular back pain is the most common complaint.
- Neurologic complaints include weakness, numbness, and paresthesias.

### *Exam*
- The most common initial findings are sensory changes, gait ataxia, and weakness.
- Ranges from nonspecific low back paraspinal tenderness to neurologic findings of myelopathy

### *Testing*
- X-rays may pick up the intradural tumor if it contains calcium
- MRI with contrast is the best imaging study to identify the tumor location and its relation to the surrounding tissues.

### *Pitfalls*
- Delay in diagnosis may be up to 2 years

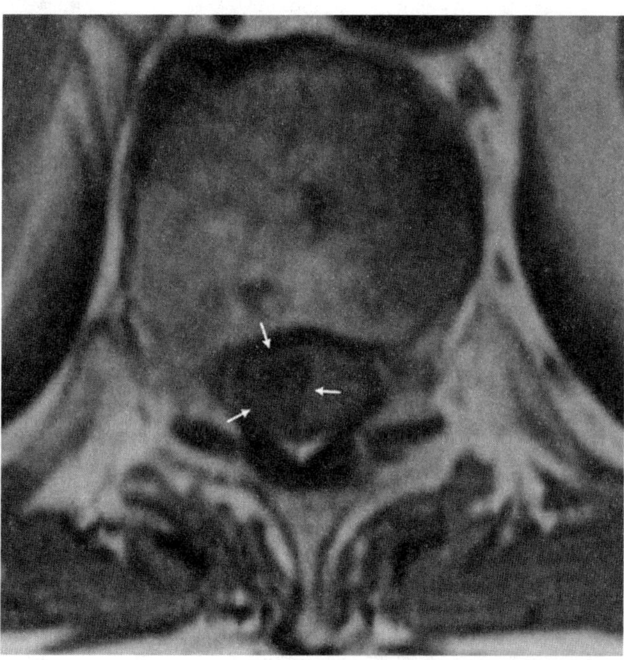

Axial thoracic T1-weighted magnetic resonance image demonstrating a large meningioma within the spinal canal (arrows). (Adapted from Fast A, Goldsher D. *Navigating the Adult Spine: Bridging Clinical Practice and Neuroradiology*. New York: Demos Medical Publishing, 2007:114.)

## Red Flags

- Spinal cord compression or myelopathy

## Treatment

### *Medical*

- Radiation therapy
- Chemotherapy

### *Exercises*

- None

### *Modalities*

- None

### *Injection*

- None

### *Surgical*

- The treatment of choice is excision of the tumor and its dural attachment.

### *Consults*

- Hematology oncology
- Radiation oncology
- Neurologic or orthopedic-spine surgery

### *Complications of treatment*

- Variable

## Prognosis

- 13% of patients can have severe functional deficits.
- Mean survival of a low-grade meningioma is 20 years.
- Mean survival of a high-grade meningioma is 12 months.
- Recurrence rate of 10%

## Helpful Hints

- Progressive neurologic decline may lead to permanent functional deficits.

## Suggested Readings

Barnholtz-Sloan JS, Kruchko C. Meningiomas: causes and risk factors. *Neurosurg Focus.* 2007;23(4):E2.

Setzer M, Vatter H, Marquardt G, Seifert V, Vrionis FD. Management of spinal meningiomas: surgical results and a review of the literature. *Neurosurg Focus.* 2007;23(4):E14.

# Meningitis

## Description

Meningitis is an infection of the meningeal lining of the central nervous system.

## Etiology/Types

- The most common bacteria are *Streptococcus pneumoniae, Haemophilus influenzae,* and *Neisseria meningitides.*
- *Staphylococcus aureus* is associated with neurosurgical procedures.
- *Staphylococcus epidermidis* is associated with ventriculoperitoneal shunts.
- Most common viral causes are *coxsackievirus, echovirus,* and *retrovirus.*
- Also caused by fungi, mycobacteria, protozoa, and spirochetes

## Epidemiology

- Annual incidence of bacterial meningitis is 5 cases per 100,000 adults per year in developed countries.
- 80% of cases of adult bacterial meningitis are caused by *Streptococcus pneumoniae* and *Neisseria meningitides.*
- Childhood meningitis is most commonly caused by *Haemophilus influenzae* B, *Streptococcus,* and *Escherichia coli.*
- Annual incidence of viral meningitis is thought to be 7.6 cases per 100,000 adults per year.

## Pathogenesis

- Results in the spread of polymorphonuclear leukocyte exudate in the subarachnoid space throughout the meninges covering the brain and spinal cord.
- Lower levels of immune cells in the subarachnoid space compared with serum concentrations allowing the organism to spread more rapidly
- Thickened fluid slows the flow of CSF, resulting in mental status changes.
- Meningitis of fungal, tuberculous, protozoan, and spirochetal origin result in slow gradual changes in mental status.

## Risk Factors

- Immunocompromised state
- Young adults

## Clinical Features

- Classic symptoms of neck stiffness, fever, and altered mental status occur in 44% of patients; 95% of these demonstrate two of the three symptoms
- In patients with bacterial meningitis:
  - 87% complain of headache
  - 83% complain of neck stiffness
  - 77% complain of fever
  - 69% had a change in cognition, nausea, vomiting, and photophobia
- Bacterial meningitis mental status changes can occur as quickly as 24 to 36 hours.
- Headache is the most common symptom of fungal meningitis.

## Natural History

- Progressive mental status changes associated with neck stiffness leading to death.

## Diagnosis

### *Differential diagnosis*

- Aseptic meningitis due to inflammatory diseases
- Brain abscess
- Epidural abscess
- Posterior fossa tumor
- Spontaneous cerebrospinal fluid leak
- Subarachnoid hemorrhage
- Subdural empyema in patients with mastoiditis or sinusitis

### *History*

- Classic triad features include neck stiffness, fever, and altered mental status.

### *Exam*

- Changes in mental status; coma
- Febrile
- Nuchal rigidity or neck stiffness is assessed by forward flexion of the neck while the patient is in a supine position (30% sensitivity, 68% specificity).
- Brudzinski's sign is positive: hip and knee flexion occur during passive neck flexion.
- Kerning's sign is positive: when the patient is in a supine position, the thigh is flexed toward the abdomen, and the patient resists knee extension.

### *Testing*

- Laboratory testing can demonstrate increased white blood cells, an increased erythrocyte sedimentation rate, and C-reactive protein.
- Lumbar spinal tap with cerebrospinal fluid culture
- Bacterial meningitis results in a turbid fluid, >1,000 white blood cells/mm$^3$, polymorphonuclear leukocytes, decreased glucose, protein level >100 mg/dl and gram-positive organisms.
- Viral meningitis results in <500 white blood cells/mm$^3$, lymphocytes, normal glucose, slightly increased protein.
- Blood cultures
- CT is used to rule out other intracranial lesions and may detect widening of subarachnoid space.

### *Pitfalls*

- Aggressive diagnosis and treatment can lead to full recovery.
- Delay in diagnosis and treatment significantly increases morbidity and mortality.

## Red Flags

- CT may be done prior to a lumbar puncture, as a sudden decrease of intracranial pressure may result in acute compression of the brainstem.

## Treatment

### *Medical*

- Due to the high potential mortality, empiric treatment and diagnostic workup should occur simultaneously.
- Intravenous antibiotics include vancomycin, penicillin, ampicillin, ceftriaxone.
- Aseptic meningitis is treated symptomatically.

### *Exercises*

- None

### *Modalities*

- None

### *Injection*

- None

### *Surgical*

- None

### *Consults*

- Infectious disease

### *Complications of treatment*

- Cerebral edema/infarction
- Seizures
- Hydrocephalus
- Hypotension
- Septic shock
- Acute respiratory distress syndrome

## Prognosis

- Aggressive diagnosis and treatment can lead to full recovery.
- Delay in diagnosis and treatment significantly increases morbidity and mortality.
- Aseptic meningitis resolves within several weeks.
- Mortality rate up to 25%

## Helpful Hints

- Due to the high potential mortality, empiric treatment and the diagnostic workup should occur simultaneously.

## Suggested Reading

Schut ES, de Gans J, van de Beek D. Community-acquired bacterial meningitis in adults. *Pract Neurol.* 2008;8(1):8–23.

# Multiple Myeloma

## Description

Multiple myeloma is a malignant neoplasm of plasma cells that can result in significant neurologic dysfunction.

## Etiology/Types

- Plasmacytoma indicates involvement of one bone.
- Multiple myeloma indicates involvement of multiple bones.

## Epidemiology

- Most common primary bone malignancy in adults
- Represents 45% of all malignant bone tumors.
- Yearly incidence is 3 to 4 cases per 100,000 individuals.
- Affects individuals from 50 to 80 years of age
- 59% involve the thoracic spine, 31% involve the lumbosacral spine, and 10% involve the cervical spine.

## Pathogenesis

- Unknown
- Multiple myeloma tends to affect highly hematopoietic bones such as the spine, ribs, skull, pelvis, and proximal ends of the humerus and femoral bones.

## Risk Factors

- Unknown

## Clinical Features

- Pain is the most common presenting complaint due to bone marrow expansion and microfractures.
- 35% of patients report low back pain.
- Pathologic fractures may occur with minimal trauma.
- Involvement of thoracic spine, ribs, and sternum may result in progressive kyphosis.
- Hypercalcemia may result in fatigue, nausea, anorexia, kidney stones, or changes in mental status.
- Increase immunoglobulin concentrations increase the risk of renal insufficiency and amyloidosis.
- Soft, gray, friable tumor that may expand from the bone into the soft tissue.
- Increased plasma cells on bone biopsy

## Natural History

- Gradual progression

## Diagnosis

### *Differential diagnosis*

- Gammopathies
- Metastasis
- Osteolytic disorders
- Plasmacytoma

### *History*

- Intermittent mild and aching pain
- Pain worsened with weight bearing and improved with recumbent positioning
- Neurologic changes later in the course of the disease

### *Exam*

- Early stages of the disease result in a normal physical examination
- With disease progression, bone tenderness, pallor, purpura, and fever predominate
- Spine and rib cage deformities
- Myelopathy

### *Testing*

- Laboratory testing may include normochromic normocytic anemia, increased leukocytes,

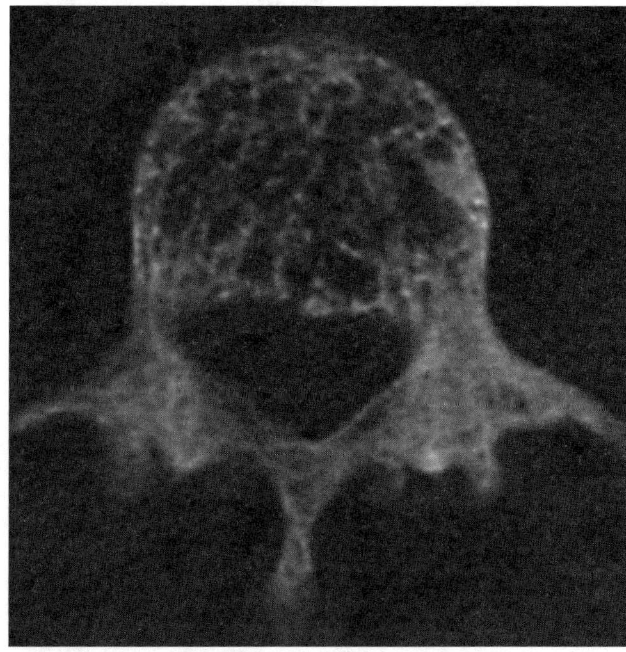

Axial thoracic computed tomography scan demonstrating multiple lytic lesions within the vertebral body characteristic of multiple myeloma. (Adapted from Fast A, Goldsher D. *Navigating the Adult Spine: Bridging Clinical Practice and Neuroradiology*. New York: Demos Medical Publishing, 2007:108.)

thrombocytopenia, a positive Coombs test, elevated erythrocyte sedimentation rate, hypercalcemia, hyperuricemia, increased creatinine.
- Impaired coagulation cascade
- Increased total serum protein concentrations including increased M proteins
- Bence-Jones proteinuria
- X-rays demonstrate characteristic osteolysis of the vertebral bodies with posterior element sparing
- CT demonstrates vertebral body involvement and the extent of bony destruction.
- MRI demonstrates changes in bone marrow.

### *Pitfalls*
- Delay in diagnosis may be >6 months.

## Red Flags
- Signs and symptoms consistent with spinal cord compression or cauda equine syndrome

## Treatment

### *Medical*
- Chemotherapy
- Radiation therapy
- Bone marrow transplantation

### *Exercises*
- Patient education
- Strengthening of the muscles surrounding the long bones
- Cardiovascular conditioning as tolerated

### *Modalities*
- None

### *Injection*
- None

### *Surgical*
- Decompressive surgery with fusion for spinal instability

### *Consults*
- Neurologic and orthopedic-spine surgery
- Radiation oncology
- Hematology oncology
- Physical medicine and rehabilitation

### *Complications of treatment*
- Spinal cord compression or cauda equina syndrome with delayed decompression

## Prognosis
- Mean survival is 3 to 5 years

## Helpful Hints
- Emergent surgical decompression for progressive spinal cord compression or cauda equina syndrome

## Suggested Readings

Bilsky MH, Azeem S. Multiple myeloma: primary bone tumor with systemic manifestations. *Neurosurg Clin N Am.* 2008;19(1):31–40.

Esteve FR, Roodman GD. Pathophysiology of myeloma bone disease. *Best Pract Res Clin Haematol.* 2007;20(4):613–624.

# Multiple Sclerosis

## Description

Multiple sclerosis is a chronic inflammatory disease affecting the central nervous system that varies in its progression and may lead to significant morbidity, including deficits in cognition, mobility, and activities of daily living.

## Etiology/Types

- Thought to be related to a viral or autoimmune mechanism
- Genetic predisposition
- Relapsing–remitting type (most common): relapses with partial or complete remissions without significant progressive deterioration.
- Primary progressive: primary deterioration with no relapses or remission
- Secondary progressive: progressive deterioration with relapsing remitting episodes
- Progressive: relapsing type

## Epidemiology

- Prevalence ranges from 40 to 220 per 100,000 in the United States.
- Prevalence increases in higher latitudes.
- Spinal cord involvement occurs in 9% to 25% of patients.
- Primary spinal cord involvement occurs in 2% to 10% of patients.
- Younger patients tend to follow a relapsing–remitting course, whereas older individuals follow a primary progressive course.

## Pathogenesis

- Multifocal demyelinated plaques are scattered throughout the central nervous system.
- Disease results in demyelization and axonal damage.
- Affects the gray and white matter

## Risk Factors

- Genetic predisposition
- Higher geographic latitudes

## Clinical Features

- Clinical diagnosis is based on two or more neurologic episodes in two or more areas of the central nervous system.
- Unilateral optic neuritis
- Diplopia
- Optic neuritis
- Sensory dysfunction
- Gait ataxia
- Spasticity
- Pain
- Neurogenic bowel or bladder dysfunction
- Fatigue
- Temperature sensitivity
- Cognitive changes

## Natural History

- The disease process begins long before the development of symptoms.

## Diagnosis

### *Differential diagnosis*

- Devic disease
- Infection
- Neoplasm
- Spinal cord infarct
- Transverse myelitis

### *History*

- Motor or sensory dysfunction
- Fatigue
- Temperature sensitivity
- Problems with balance and gait

### *Exam*

- Positive Lhermitte's sign
- Motor deficits
- Gait ataxia
- Neurogenic bowel or bladder dysfunction
- Disability is measured using Kurtzke's expanded disability status scale ranging from 0.0 (normal) to 10.0 (death).

### *Testing*

- Laboratory testing demonstrates oligoclonal bands or IgG within the CSF.
- MRI is used for diagnosis and demonstrates "plaque-like" lesions of increased signal on T2-weighted images within the spinal cord or brain.
  - Preference for dorsolateral aspect of the spinal cord
- Dawson's fingers are the characteristic lesions surrounding the deep veins of the brain.

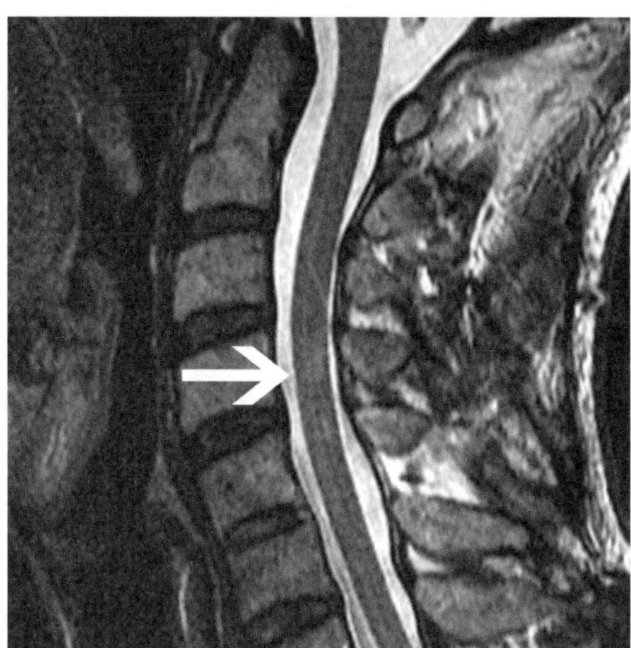

Sagittal cervical T2-weighted magnetic resonance image demonstrating minimal increased signal within the spinal cord at the C4–C5 level (arrow) resulting from multiple sclerosis.

- 48% of patients have positive findings in the cervical spinal cord.
- Visual and auditory evoked potentials
- Somatosensory evoked potentials

### *Pitfalls*
- Delay in diagnosis

## Red Flags
- Progressive neurologic decline
- Bowel or bladder dysfunction

## Treatment

### *Medical*
- Intravenous (IV) methylprednisolone 1,000 mg for 3 days, which helps to speed recovery during an acute exacerbation
- Disease-modifying drugs have been shown to be effective, primarily against the relapsing–remitting type.
- Interferon β-1b, interferon β-1a, glatiramer acetate, mitoxantrone
- Symptomatic treatment is directed at neurogenic bladder, fatigue, heat intolerance, spasms, pain, cognition and mood, speech, and swallowing.
- Avoidance of increased environmental temperatures, which results in increased fatigue and weakness

### *Exercises*
- General strengthening at a moderate intensity in colder temperatures
- Endurance training at a low or moderate intensity
- Pool therapy
- Stretching

### *Modalities*
- Heat, cold, ultrasound, and transcutaneous electrical nerve stimulation have been used for symptomatic relief of local pain and muscle spasms.

### *Injection*
- None

### *Surgical*
- None

### *Consults*
- Neurology

### *Complications of treatment*
- Patients may develop neutralizing antibodies to the medications within 2 years, decreasing their effectiveness. If no antibodies develop there is no concern about antibody development thereafter.

## Prognosis
- Variable
- Spinal cord plaques found on MRI correlate with the degree of disability.
- Median time from symptoms onset until use of a cane is 20 years.
- Median time from symptoms onset until use of a wheelchair is 30 years.
- 50% of patients will need assistance ambulating within 15 years after onset.
- Unknown how well the medications reduce disability

## Helpful Hints
- Global assessment is important due to the diffuse involvement of the central nervous system.

## Suggested Reading
Noseworthy JH, Lucchinetti C, Rodriguez M, Weinshenker BG. Multiple sclerosis. *N Engl J Med*. 2000;343(13):938–952.

# Myofascial Pain Syndrome

## Description

Myofascial pain syndrome is a regional pain disorder characterized by a localized hyperirritable and hypersensitive palpable area within a taut band of skeletal muscle or muscle fascia that refers pain in a distal nondermatomal distribution when compressed.

## Etiology/Types

- Unknown

## Epidemiology

- Occurs in 30% of patients in a general medical clinic and up to 93% of patients referred to a pain clinic
- Latent trigger points are trigger points that are tender to palpation, which may be associated with stiffness and decreased range of motion that is not associated with complaints of pain.
- Active trigger points are trigger points associated with pain complaints.

## Pathogenesis

- Myofascial trigger points produce motor changes, sensory hyperalgesia and dysesthesias, and autonomic symptoms that include salivation, changes in skin temperature, sweating, and proprioceptive changes.
- The local twitch response is a brisk contraction of muscle fibers in a taut band that is elicited by snapping palpation or the insertion of a needle that is thought to correlate with an increased density of sensory receptors and spontaneous electrical activity close to motor endplates.
- Sustained release of acetylcholine at the motor end plates with sustained muscle contraction and local ischemia results in the release of inflammatory substances causing muscle pain.
- Spinal segmental sensitization may develop if myofascial pain is left untreated.

## Risk Factors

- Anxiety
- Chronic infection
- Chronic muscle imbalance
- Degenerative joint disease
- Nerve root compression or irritation
- Nutritional deficiencies
- Poor posture or ergonomics
- Repetitive strain injuries or repetitive microtrauma
- Scoliosis
- Sleep deprivation
- Thyroid disorders
- Traumatic injury

## Clinical Features

- Sudden onset
- Pain in a distributed pattern
- Restricted joint range of motion with increased sensitivity to stretching
- Muscle weakness due to pain with no muscular atrophy
- Palpation of the painful site resulting in a reproduction of the characteristic pain
- A palpable muscle band with a local twitch response

## Natural History

- General worsening of pain complaints

## Diagnosis

### *Differential diagnosis*

- Chronic pain syndrome
- Fibromyalgia
- Fracture
- Infection
- Joint osteoarthritis
- Neoplasm
- Psychological disorders
- Polymyalgia rheumatica
- Polymyositis
- Radiculopathy

### *History*

- Localized or regional deep aching pain
- Pain intensity ranges from mild to severe.
- Stiff joints
- Fatigue/weakness
- Sleep difficulty
- Parasthesias
- Numbness

### *Exam*

- Posture asymmetry
- Active and passive range of motion restrictions
- Abnormal movement patterns
- Palpation of trigger point
- The trigger point often has a "ropelike" consistency

### Testing

- Algometry as described by Fischer
- Imaging can be used to rule out other conditions.

### Pitfalls

- Often underdiagnosed and undertreated
- Unemployment, poor coping ability, and constant pain are related to poor treatment.

## Red Flags

- Fracture
- Neoplasm
- Neurologic deficits
- Infection

## Treatment

### Medical

- Acetaminophen
- Muscle relaxants
- NSAIDs
- Analgesics
- Dry needling

### Exercises

- The use of vapocoolant spray over the entire trigger point region and reference zone followed by passive muscle stretching
- Progressive stretching and strengthening

### Modalities

- Heat, cold, ultrasound, and transcutaneous electrical nerve stimulation have been used for symptomatic relief of pain and muscle spasms.
- Massage
- Ischemic compression

### Injection

- Trigger point injections with the trigger point stabilized between the thumb and forefinger using local anesthetic [procaine (higher risk of anaphylaxis) or lidocaine], which decreases local soreness
- A local twitch response is critical for immediate relief of muscle tightness and pain.
- Corticosteroids, saline, and botulinum toxin have also been used in injections.
- Paraspinous block with local anesthetic

### Surgical

- None

### Consults

- None

### Complications of treatment

- Trigger point injections have a low risk of complications, which include bleeding, infection, allergic reaction to the injected medications.

## Prognosis

- Few studies have been completed that demonstrate patients are able to increase their coping skills and life satisfaction while decreasing sick time.

## Helpful Hints

- Generally underdiagnosed and undertreated

## Suggested Reading

Borg-Stein J, Simons DG. Focused review: myofascial pain. *Arch Phys Med Rehabil.* 2002;83(3 Suppl 1):S40–S47, S48–S49.

# Neck Pain Associated with Occupation

## Description

Acute or chronic neck pain associated with occupational activities. Also known as repetitive strain injury (RSI), cumulative trauma disorder (CTD), occupational cervicobrachial disorder (OCD), and work-related musculoskeletal disorder (WMSD).

## Etiology/Types

- Neck pain probably arises from a combination of individual and workplace factors.

## Epidemiology

- Prevalence of neck pain in workers ranges from 27% to 49%.
- 11% to 14% of workers annually are limited in activities due to neck pain.
- The highest prevalence of occupational neck pain is found in office and hospital workers.
- The lowest prevalence of occupational neck pain is found in forest and industrial workers.

## Pathogenesis

- Excess shoulder girdle muscles loading
- Muscle strains are considered unlikely with computer use as there is less than 5% of maximal voluntary contraction.
- Increased cervical pain is associated with decreased cervical rotation and increased activity in the superficial cervical flexors with an associated compensatory decreased activity in the deep cervical flexors.
- Muscle biopsy results note increased fiber cross-sectional areas and mitochondrial disturbances of type 1 fibers.
- Increased inflammatory mediators have been found in local muscles that correlate with pain.

## Risk Factors

- Female gender
- Forceful exertions
- High job demands
- High level static contractions
- Increasing age, particularly in the fourth and fifth decade of life
- Low physical capacity
- Previous musculoskeletal pain
- Poor social support at work
- Poor work posture
- Poor workstation ergonomics
- Prolonged static loads and extreme postures
- Repetitive job tasks
- Sedentary job activities

## Clinical Features

- Neck pain without symptoms in the lower extremities

## Natural History

- Variable

## Diagnosis

### *Differential diagnosis*

- Infection
- Osteoarthritis
- Radiculopathy
- Referred pain from cardiothoracic structures
- Tumor

### *History*

- Increased pain, tiredness, and stiffness
- Pain worse during workday and improved during weekend
- Sleep difficulty
- Associated headaches

### *Exam*

- Poor posture/head forward posture
- Decreased cervical range of motion, particularly with rotation
- Increased muscle tension in the upper trapezii, levator scapulae, and scalenes
- Tenderness to palpation of the superior nuchal line

### *Testing*

- Plain radiographs may demonstrate loss of the normal lordotic curve suggesting spasm.
- Magnetic resonance imaging may be used to rule out soft tissue pathology.
- Electrodiagnostic studies can be used to assess for radiculopathy.

### *Pitfalls*

- Overlooking workplace and psychological factors

## Red Flags

- Weakness, numbness, or tingling

- Acute pain and muscle spasm that may be associated with a fracture.

## Treatment

### *Medical*

- Cognitive behavioral therapy
- Ergonomic interventions have not been shown to prevent neck pain in the literature, although a thorough discussion may uncover poor workstation ergonomics that can be easily altered.
- Analgesics
- NSAIDs
- Acupuncture has been described to be helpful for symptomatic relief.

### *Exercises*

- Exercise program focusing on motor relearning training
- Manipulation
- Mobilization

### *Modalities*

- Heat, cold, ultrasound, and transcutaneous electrical nerve stimulation have been used for symptomatic relief of pain and muscle spasms.

### *Injection*

- Trigger point injections for symptoms of myofascial pain
- Cervical epidural steroid injections for radicular symptoms have been shown to provide short-term symptomatic relief.
- Zygapophyseal (facet) joint injections and radiofrequency neurotomy have been shown to provide pain relief.

### *Surgical*

- Surgical decompression for radicular symptoms can produce rapid and significant symptom relief.
- Percutaneous or open surgical treatment of neck pain without radicular symptoms lacks evidence.

### *Consults*

- Psychology or psychiatry
- Physical medicine and rehabilitation
- Neurologic or orthopedic-spine surgery for surgical indications

### *Complications of treatment*

- Less than 1% of cervical epidural steroid injections result in serious adverse reactions.
- 4% of open surgical procedures in the cervical spine can result in serious adverse reactions.

## Prognosis

- 60% to 80% of workers with neck will continue to have neck pain one year later.
- Workers with little influence over their job situation have a slightly poorer prognosis.
- General exercise is associated with a better prognosis.
- Less than half of patients with neck and shoulder pain will be free of pain after 1 to 5 years.

## Helpful Hints

- Review posture and workstation ergonomics
- Review the use of heavy shoulder bags

## Suggested Reading

Andersen JH, Kaergaard A, Frost P, et al. Physical, psychosocial, and individual risk factors for neck/shoulder pain with pressure tenderness in the muscles among workers performing monotonous, repetitive work. *Spine*. 2002;27(6):660–667.

# Neck Pain in Athletes

## Description

Neck pain in athletes encompasses mild to serious cervical injuries.

## Etiology/Types

- Cervical strain or sprain
- Overuse injuries
- Cervical degenerative disc disease with or without radiculopathy
- Cervical spinal cord neurapraxia
- Stingers or burners
- Cervical compression/spinous process fractures
- Blunt trauma to the carotid artery

## Epidemiology

- Sporting activities are the second most common cause of neck pain after motor vehicle accidents presenting in the emergency department.
- Most commonly related to high-velocity contact sports
- Cervical strains and sprains are the most common injury.

## Pathogenesis

- Strains occur as eccentric stretch injuries within the substance or musculotendinous junction of the muscle
- Sprains involve a stretch injury to ligamentous structures.
- Spinous process fractures can occur from a strong muscle contraction.
- Cervical compression fractures are primarily due to hyperflexion.
- Blunt trauma to the carotid artery may cause dissection, thrombus, or emboli.

## Risk Factors

- Football, hockey, wrestling, gymnastics
- Older age
- Preexisting spinal stenosis (cervical cord <13 mm in the sagittal diameter) may predispose athletes to cervical spinal cord injury.
- Spear tackling in football causes a loss of the normal protective cervical lordosis increasing risk of bony or neurologic injury.

## Clinical Features

- Clinical features are based on the mechanism of injury.



## Natural History

- Variable

## Diagnosis

### Differential diagnosis

- Acute cholecystitis
- Benign or neoplastic neck mass
- Carotid or aortic dissection
- Gastroesophageal reflux
- Occipital neuralgia
- Pharyngitis
- Referred pain from cardiopulmonary disease
- Sternoclavicular arthritis or sprain
- Superior vena cava syndrome

### History

- Important to first assess airway, breathing, circulation, level of consciousness, and apprehension
- Need to determine if neck pain is isolated to the anterior, lateral, or posterior regions.
- Neurologic symptoms or deficits
- Balance or gait abnormalities
- Bowel or bladder dysfunction

### Exam

- Assess midline cervical tenderness, presence of static cervical pain or cervical pain with active range of motion, severe cervical rigidity, or neurologic deficits
- Lhermitte's sign
- Spurling's test
- Shoulder and scapulothoracic articulation

### Testing

- X-rays of the cervical spine with >3.5 mm of displacement between flexion and extension views or 11 degrees of rotation on an anterioposterior view indicates ligamentous laxity.
- MRI is used for assessing cervical spinal cord injury or ligamentous injuries.
- CT is used to better delineate bony anatomy.

### Pitfalls

- Passive range of motion should not be done on patients with a potential cervical cord injury
- Missing associated ligamentous injury with a cervical compression fracture

## Red Flags

- Unconscious athletes are assumed to have cervical spinal cord injury until proven otherwise
- Witnessed spear tackling using the head may result in a spinal cord injury
- Severe cervical spasm
- Athlete apprehension
- Cervical pain with active range or motion

## Treatment

### Medical

- If there is a possibility for a cervical injury, the neck needs to be immobilized with further workup in a nearby emergency room.
- Cervical cord neurapraxia should be treated as a severe spinal cord injury.
- Oral corticosteroids or NSAIDs for cervical radiculopathy
- Compression fractures may be treated with a semi-rigid cervical collar for 8 to 10 weeks.
- Spinous process fractures require a cervical collar for 4 to 6 weeks.

### Exercises

- Gentle range-of-motion exercises for most cervical strains, degenerative disc disease, or radiculopathy
- Isometric strengthening
- Sports-specific exercises or drills

### Modalities

- Heat, cold, ultrasound, and transcutaneous electrical nerve stimulation have been used for symptomatic relief of pain and muscle spasms.

### Injection

- Epidural steroid injections for radicular symptoms

### Surgical

- Indications for surgery include persistent or recurrent radicular symptoms, cervical myelopathy, and progressive neurologic deficit.
- Stable one-level cervical fusions at C3 or below is not a contraindication for return to contact sports.
- Two or three level cervical fusions without neurologic deficits should avoid contact sports.
- More than a three-level fusion or a fusion above C3 is an absolute contraindication for return to contact sports.

### Consults

- Physical medicine and rehabilitation
- Neurologic or orthopedic-spine surgery

### Complications of treatment

- Persistent spinal cord injury

## Prognosis

- Return to sport following a cervical sprain or strain occurs when the athlete meets the following 3 criteria:
  - Is pain free
  - Can demonstrate full strength and range of motion
  - Has regained sports-specific neck function

## Helpful Hints

- Unconscious athletes are assumed to have cervical spinal cord injury until proven otherwise.

## Suggested Reading

Zmurko MG, Tannoury TY, Tannoury CA. Cervical sprains, disc herniations, minor fractures, and other cervical injuries in the athlete. *Clin Sports Med.* 2003;22(3):513–521.

# Neck Strain

## Description

A neck strain results from an injury to the dynamic muscle stabilizers or static ligamentous structures of the neck.

## Etiology/Types

- May be associated with mechanical overload or a prolonged abnormal posture

## Epidemiology

- Chronic strain or acute or repetitive neck injuries make up 85% of all neck pain complaints.

## Pathogenesis

- May be related to ligamentous or muscular injury from excessive tension or stretching
- Muscle fatigue from overuse
- Muscle spasm caused by muscle overload
- Paraspinal muscle deconditioning due to previous injury

## Risk Factors

- Mechanical overload
- Muscle overuse
- Prolonged abnormal posture

## Clinical Features

- Localized or diffuse nonradiating neck pain
- Worsened with abnormal posture
- May be associated with headaches

## Natural History

- Usually a self-limiting condition
- Recurrent episodes of increasing frequency and intensity are possible.

## Diagnosis

### *Differential diagnosis*

- Herniated nucleus pulposus
- Klippel–Feil syndrome describes patients with a congenital fusion of two vertebral bodies, several vertebral bodies, or the entire cervical spine.
- Occipital neuralgia
- Osteoarthritis
- Posterior element fractures
- Soft tissue or bony trauma
- Spondyloarthropathies
- Temporomandibular joint abnormalities with referral into the neck
- Tumors
- Torticollis

### *History*

- Diffuse or localized tenderness with possible radiation into the shoulders, scapular region, occipital region, or anterior chest wall
- Pain with neck range of motion
- Worsens with activity and improved with recumbency
- Dull, aching pain

### *Exam*

- Normal neurologic examination
- Tenderness to palpation of paraspinal muscles
- Decreased neck range of motion

### *Testing*

- Laboratory tests are usually normal.
- Plain radiographs are usually normal, although there may be enough muscle spasm to result in loss of the normal cervical lordosis.
- Congenital abnormalities are rare in the cervical spine.
- Unless indicated, advanced imaging studies will not clarify the diagnosis.

### *Pitfalls*

- Lack of correlation of the history to the physical examination
- Overlooking a neoplasm

## Red Flags

- Neurologic changes
- Soft tissue or bony abnormalities may be an early sign of fracture or neoplasm.
- Skin rashes suggest a systemic illness.

## Treatment

### *Medical*

- NSAIDs
- Muscle relaxants
- Short-term opioids
- Limited use of a cervical collar, primarily at night
- Acupuncture has been described as helpful for symptomatic relief.

### Exercises

- Minimal or no bed rest
- Intermittent lightweight cervical traction to decrease spasms and pain
- Physical activity within the patient's pain tolerance
- Physical therapy with a home exercise program focused on pain control and regaining mobility

### Modalities

- Heat, cold, ultrasound, and transcutaneous electrical nerve stimulation have been used for symptomatic relief of pain and muscle spasms.

### Injection

- Trigger point injections to block the reflexive spasm if 2 to 4 weeks have passed without significant improvement.

### Surgical

- Surgical intervention is possible for unstable spine.

### Consults

- Physical medicine and rehabilitation
- Neurologic or orthopedic-spine surgeon, if trauma was involved.

### Complications of treatment

- Variable

## Prognosis

- Excellent chance of recovery over several weeks
- Pain may continue for months or years.

## Helpful Hints

- Generally a self-limiting condition
- The physician should reassure the patient that no damage will occur with continued activity.

## Suggested Readings

Foye PM, Sullivan WJ, Sable AW, Panagos A, Zuhosky JP, Irwin RW. Industrial medicine and acute musculoskeletal rehabilitation. 3. Work-related musculoskeletal conditions: the role for physical therapy, occupational therapy, bracing, and modalities. *Arch Phys Med Rehabil.* 2007;88 (3 Suppl 1):S14–S17.

Swezey RL. Chronic neck pain. *Rheum Dis Clin North Am.* 1996;22(3):411–437.

# Neurofibroma

## Description

Neurofibroma is a common autosomal dominant syndrome of the central and peripheral nervous systems.

## Etiology/Types

- Neurofibromatosis type I (peripheral neurofibromatosis) is the most common hereditary neoplastic syndrome, which is associated with a chromosome 17 defect.
- Neurofibromatosis type II, which is associated with acoustic neuromas, is due to a chromosome 22 defect.

## Epidemiology

- Incidence is 1 in 3,000 live births.
- Occurs in adults aged 30 to 60 years.

## Pathogenesis

- Arises from Schwann cells, fibroblasts, and nerve fibers
- 41% of cases affect the thoracic spine, 31% affect the lumbar spine, 26% affect the cervical spine, and 2% affect the sacrum.
- Can involve the sensory, motor, or combined sensorimotor portions of the nerve

## Risk Factors

- Genetic predisposition

## Clinical Features

- Clinical findings include neurofibromas, lisch nodules, café-au-lait spots, freckling, optic gliomas, and skeletal dysplasia.
- Adults typically present with kyphoscoliosis.
- A small number of patients may have no spinal abnormalities.

## Natural History

- 3% of patients have malignant transformation.
- Malignant transformation is more likely in patients with multiple lesions.

## Diagnosis

### *Differential diagnosis*

- Meningioma
- Schwannoma

### *History*

- The initial presenting symptom is axial, radicular, or referred pain.
- Worsened with recumbent positioning, sneezing, or a Valsalva maneuver

### *Exam*

- Motor, sensory, and reflex changes may be noted.
- Possible asymmetric signs of spinal cord injury may be present.
- Spastic motor loss

### *Testing*

- X-rays may demonstrate erosion of the pedicle, intervertebral foramen widening, or vertebral scalloping.
- Scoliosis occurs in 17% of patients.
- Normal X-rays are consistent with an intradural tumor.
- MRI may note multiple intradural and extramedullary masses

### *Pitfalls*

- Delay in diagnosis may range from 1 to 4 years.

## Red Flags

- Signs of spinal cord compression

## Treatment

### *Medical*

- Supportive

### *Exercises*

- General conditioning exercises to prevent deconditioning

### *Modalities*

- None

### *Injection*

- None

### *Surgical*

- Surgical resection is preferred for spinal cord or nerve root compression.
- Resection is difficult with multiple lesions or intimacy with vital structures.

### *Consults*

- Physical medicine and rehabilitation
- Neurologic or orthopedic-spine surgery
- Neurology

*Complications of treatment*

- Peripheral nerve injury
- Spinal cord injury
- Complications related to surgery

## Prognosis

- Based on location of masses

## Helpful Hints

- Important to assess for peripheral signs associated with neurofibromatosis

## Suggested Readings

Crawford AH, Parikh S, Schorry EK, Von Stein D. The immature spine in type-1 neurofibromatosis. *J Bone Joint Surg Am.* 2007;89 (Suppl 1):123–142.

Ferner RE. Neurofibromatosis 1 and neurofibromatosis 2: a twenty first century perspective. *Lancet Neurol.* 2007;6(4):340–351.

Savar A, Cestari DM. Neurofibromatosis type I: genetics and clinical manifestations. *Semin Ophthalmol.* 2008;23(1):45–51.

# Osteoblastoma

## Description

Osteoblastoma is a rare, benign neoplasm of bone most commonly found in the lumbar spine.

## Etiology/Types

- Unknown

## Epidemiology

- Most common in individuals up to 30 years of age
- 3% of all benign bone tumors
- Male to female ratio is 2.5:1
- Most common in the axial spine
- 50% of cases affect the lumbar spine.
- 38% of cases affect the cervical spine.

## Pathogenesis

- Unknown

## Risk Factors

- Unknown

## Clinical Features

- Tumors tend to be 2 to 10 cm in length and made up of well-circumscribed hemorrhagic granular tissue
- Average duration of symptoms before diagnosis is 14 months.
- Insidious localized dull, aching pain overlying the involved bony segment
- Possible torticollis with cervical involvement
- Formation of scoliosis with thoracic or lumbar involvement
- Possible radicular pain associated with lumbar involvement
- Mass may encircle nerve roots

## Natural History

- Progressive enlargement

## Diagnosis

### *Differential diagnosis*

- Giant cell tumor
- Hyperparathyroidism
- Osteoid osteoma
- Osteosarcoma

### *History*

- Insidious localized dull, aching pain
- Pain worsens with activity
- Scoliosis

### *Exam*

- Characteristic localized tenderness with mild swelling over the involved spinal segment
- Increased pain with extension of the spine
- Neurologic findings associated with compression of the nerve roots or spinal cord
- Positive straight leg raise has been found in 25% of patients
- Muscle atrophy may be noted adjacent to the tumor

### *Testing*

- X-rays tend to be nonspecific; most common location is in the posterior elements with rare involvement of the vertebral body.
- Rarely found to affect the atlas and axis

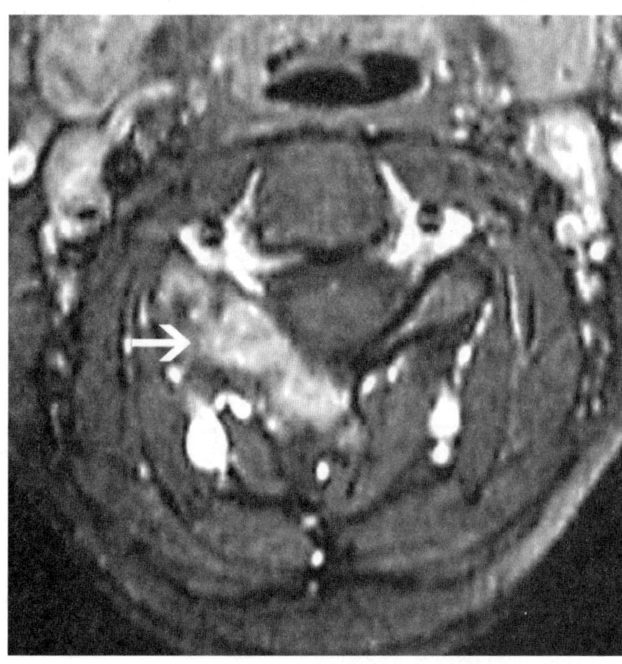

Axial cervical T1-weighted magnetic resonance image with contrast and fat suppression demonstrating an osteoblastoma expanding into the right lamina (arrow). (Adapted from Fast A, Goldsher D. *Navigating the Adult Spine: Bridging Clinical Practice and Neuroradiology.* New York: Demos Medical Publishing, 2007:113.)

- The mass tends to appear as a well-circumscribed lesion with a thin layer of bone surrounding a radiolucent or opaque center.
- Bone scan may be helpful in identifying a lesion that does not appear on X-rays
- CT allows for assessment of the extent of bony tumor penetration
- MRI allows for visualization of tumor penetration into the adjacent soft tissue.
- MRI with contrast is used periodically for focal enhancement of the mass.

### *Pitfalls*

- Delay in diagnosis of months to years

## Red Flags

- Progressive radiculopathy
- Spinal cord compression

## Treatment

### *Medical*

- Radiation therapy for lesions that cannot be completely excised
- Radiation therapy may result in malignant transformation, increased spinal cord compression, or necrosis.
- Chemotherapy has been found to slow the growth of the mass.

### *Exercises*

- None

### *Modalities*

- None

### *Injection*

- None

### *Surgical*

- Surgical excision of the tumor mass is the preferred method of treatment.
- Partial curettage is used for masses that are inaccessible for full excision.

### *Consults*

- Neurologic or orthopedic-spine surgery
- Radiation oncology

### *Complications of treatment*

- Radiation therapy may result in malignant transformation, increased spinal cord compression, or necrosis

## Prognosis

- Benign course
- Involvement of the axial spine is associated with greater morbidity and mortality.
- Pain resolves with complete excision.
- 5% recurrence rate
- Recurrence may occur up to 17 years.

## Helpful Hints

- Benign slow growing lesion
- Nerve root or spinal cord compression is possible.

## Suggested Readings

Kan P, Schmidt MH. Osteoid osteoma and osteoblastoma of the spine. *Neurosurg Clin N Am*. 2008;19(1):65–70.

Zileli M, Cagli S, Basdemir G, Ersahin Y. Osteoid osteomas and osteoblastomas of the spine. *Neurosurg Focus*. 2003;15(5):E5.

# Osteochondroma

## Description

Osteochondroma is a common benign tumor of bone that may occur in a solitary location or in multiple locations.

## Etiology/Types

- Thought to be related to abnormal cartilage growth during skeletal immaturity, which ceases growth once skeletal maturity has been reached

## Epidemiology

- Makes up 36% of all benign bone tumors.
- 60% of patients are aged 30 or under, although it has been reported in older patients.
- Multiple lesions develop in patients before 20 years of age.
- Male to female ratio is 2:1

## Pathogenesis

- Thought to be caused by a defect in the periosteal bone of the epiphyseal plate during embryogenesis

## Risk Factors

- Unknown

## Clinical Features

- Mild pain related to mechanical irritation of adjacent soft tissues
- Progression of pain over years
- Continued growth may result in decreased joint range of motion and function
- May result in scoliosis, radiculopathy, spinal stenosis, or cord compression

## Natural History

- Stops growing at skeletal maturity and is frequently asymptomatic, although with continued growth, it may lead to progressive neurologic compromise.
- Horner's syndrome
- Brown-Séquard syndrome
- Sudden death
- Spinal cord injury
- Nerve root injury
- Occlusion of the vertebral artery
- Hoarseness
- Dysphagia

## Diagnosis

### Differential diagnosis

- Callus associated with fracture
- Chondroblastomas
- Chondroid metaplasia
- Chondromas
- Malignant transformation
- Osteophytes

### History

- Mild, deep pain
- Pain improved with rest and worsened with activity
- Painless palpable bony mass
- Decreased joint range of motion
- Possible motor, sensory, reflex changes
- Possible bowel or bladder incontinence

### Exam

- May demonstrate no neurologic deficit, although there may be significant neurologic deficits associated with the level of involvement.
- Tenderness with palpation of the mass
- Decreased joint or segment range of motion

### Testing

- X-rays can be diagnostic, demonstrating protrusion of the mass on a sessile or bony stalk arising from the bone.
- May be an incidental finding on X-rays of an asymptomatic patient
- Bone scan demonstrates increased uptake at the site of the tumor
- CT is used to demonstrate the size and location of the tumor and its relation to the bony and soft tissue structures.
- MRI is not good at imaging the bony structure.

### Pitfalls

- Patients should be monitored for changes in symptomatology or tumor size.

## Red Flags

- Signs and symptoms of nerve root or spinal cord compression, which includes tetraparesis

## Treatment

### Medical

- None

### *Exercises*

- None

### *Modalities*

- None

### *Injection*

- None

### *Surgical*

- Surgical decompression is required if there is neurologic compromise.

### *Consults*

- Neurologic or orthopedic-spine surgery

### *Complications of treatment*

- Complications related to surgery

## Prognosis

- Resolution of pain noted with surgical excision
- Patients should be monitored as osteochondromas may become malignant.

## Helpful Hints

- Monitoring patients for changes in the signs and symptoms of a symptomatic tumor

## Suggested Readings

Cooke RS, Cumming WJ, Cowie RA. Osteochondroma of the cervical spine: case report and review of the literature. *Br J Neurosurg.* 1994;8(3):359–363.

Gille O, Pointillart V, Vital JM. Course of spinal solitary osteochondromas. *Spine.* 2005;30(1):E13–E19.

Giudicissi-Filho M, de Holanda CV, Borba LA, Rassi-Neto A, Ribeiro CA, de Oliveira JG. Cervical spinal cord compression due to an osteochondroma in hereditary multiple exostosis: case report and review of the literature. *Surg Neurol.* 2006;66 (Suppl 3):S7–S11.

# Osteogenesis Imperfecta

## Description

Osteogenesis imperfecta is a genetic disorder of connective tissue that results in decreased bone mass resulting in bony fragility.

## Etiology/Types

- Type I: mild form, dominant inheritable form, most common
- Type II: lethal form resulting in perinatal death
- Type III: severe progressive form resulting in scoliosis and a short stature
- Type IV: moderate form
- Type V: variable severity, which may include radial head dislocation and interosseous calcification
- Type VI: moderate form
- Type VII: moderate to severe form, may result in intrauterine fractures

## Epidemiology

- Prevalence is up to 1 in 5,000 individuals.

## Pathogenesis

- Abnormal collagen maturation due to mutation of the two genes that encode collagen type 1 alpha chains (*COL1A1* and *COL1A2*)
- Type I is autosomal dominant.

## Risk Factors

- Genetic predisposition

## Clinical Features

- Type I is associated with blue sclera, short to normal stature, variable bone fragility, and hearing loss.
- Bone fragility increases in the following order: type I < types IV, V, VI, VII < type III < type II.
- Short stature is the result of multiple fractures, bowing of the long bones, and kyphoscoliosis.
- 80% of individuals develop scoliosis.
- Ligamentous laxity
- Otosclerosis
- Premature vascular calcification
- Constipation
- Easy bruisability
- Discoloration of teeth
- Micrognathia
- Temporal bulging

## Natural History

- Multiple fractures
- Progressive scoliosis

## Diagnosis

### *Differential diagnosis*

- Achondrogenesis
- Battered child syndrome
- Idiopathic juvenile osteoporosis
- Steroid-induced osteoporosis

### *History*

- Back pain due to vertebral body fractures and associated muscle spasm

### *Exam*

- Blue sclera
- Bony tenderness with associated muscle spasm
- Scoliosis
- Limb abnormalities due to previous fractures

### *Testing*

- X-rays note diffuse osteopenia with flattened vertebral bodies, "fish" vertebrae, and anterior wedging of the vertebral bodies.

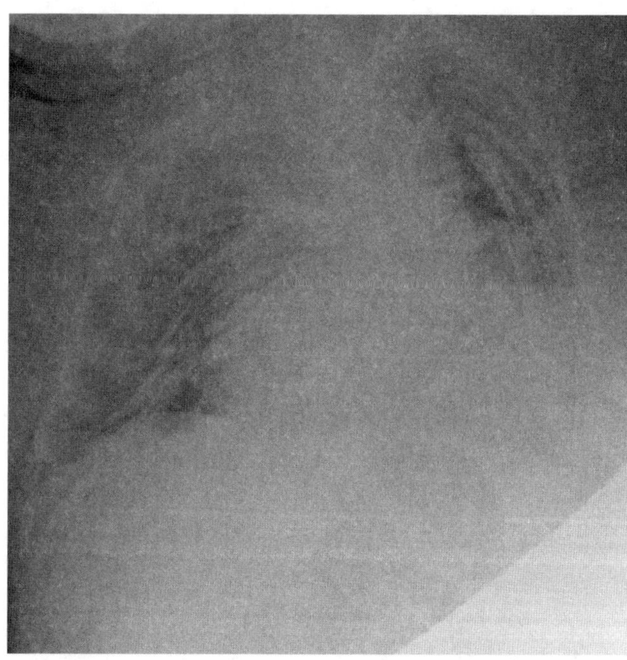

Posterioanterior chest plain radiograph demonstrating scoliosis and diffuse osteopenia characteristic in osteogenesis imperfecta. (Courtesy of Keith Hentel, MD.)

- Radiographic evidence of six or more biconcave vertebrae prior to puberty indicates the progressive development of severe (>50-degree angle) scoliosis.
- CT and MRI may be useful in assessing for suspected vertebral body fractures not evident on plain radiographs.

### Pitfalls

- Missed vertebral body fracture

## Red Flags

- Missed vertebral body fracture

## Treatment

### Medical

- NSAIDs and analgesics for pain
- Intravenous pamidronate may be used to treat decreased bone density and pain.
- Bracing does not prevent the progression of scoliosis.

### Exercises

- Focus on maximizing mobility and functional activities, although this can be severely limited in patients with severe bone fragility.
- Exercise does not prevent the progression of scoliosis.

### Modalities

- Heat, cold, ultrasound, and transcutaneous electrical nerve stimulation have been used for symptomatic relief of pain and muscle spasms.

### Injection

- None

### Surgical

- Percutaneous vertebral augmentation for vertebral body-compression fractures
- Spinal fusion for scoliosis >50 degrees to halt the loss in pulmonary function

### Consults

- Neurologic or orthopedic-spine surgery
- Rheumatology

### Complications of treatment

- Complication rates approach 50% with surgical management of scoliosis.

## Prognosis

- Pulmonary compromise is the primary cause of death in patients with a thoracic scoliosis of 60 degrees or greater.

## Helpful Hints

- Focus on maximizing mobility and functional activities

## Suggested Readings

Engelbert RH, Pruijs HE, Beemer FA, Helders PJ. Osteogenesis imperfecta in childhood: treatment strategies. *Arch Phys Med Rehabil.* 1998;79(12):1590–1594.

Rauch F, Glorieux FH. Osteogenesis imperfecta. *Lancet.* 2004;363(9418):1377–1385.

# Osteoid Osteoma

## Description

Osteoid osteoma is a painful, benign primary bone tumor.

## Etiology/Types

- Unknown

## Epidemiology

- Makes up 12% of all benign tumors.
- Most common between the ages of 20 and 30 years
- 18% are located in the axial spine.
- 44% of these affect the lumbar spine and 30% affect the cervical and thoracic spines.
- Male to female ratio is 2:1

## Pathogenesis

- Theories include a consequence of a chronic infection or reparative process or a benign bone neoplasm with limited growth potential.

## Risk Factors

- Unknown

## Clinical Features

- Pain that is relieved with aspirin or NSAIDs is the characteristic feature, although some osteoid osteomas may not be painful or may not respond to anti-inflammatory drugs.
- An initial manifestation may be scoliosis.
- Osteoid osteoma of the cervical spine is only found in the pedicles and the posterior elements.
- Cervical presentation may include torticollis and occipital headache.
- 75% of presentations occur in the neural arch, 18% occur at the zygapophyseal (facet) joints, and 7% occur in the vertebral body.

## Natural History

- Generally described as increasing pain
- Irreversible scoliosis

## Diagnosis

### *Differential diagnosis*

- Eosinophilic granuloma
- Ewing's sarcoma
- Fracture
- Herniated nucleus pulposis
- Lumbar strain
- Metastasis
- Osteoblastoma
- Osteomyelitis
- Osteosarcoma

### *History*

- Vague intermittent pain with increasing intensity
- Pain characteristically improved with aspirin or NSAIDs.
- Pain is worse at night.
- Pain not improved with heat or rest.
- Possible radicular symptoms

### *Exam*

- Tenderness over the involved bony structure
- A progressive scoliosis may be related to asymmetrical muscle spasm.
- Superficial presentation may result in swelling and erythema.
- Sensory changes are rare.

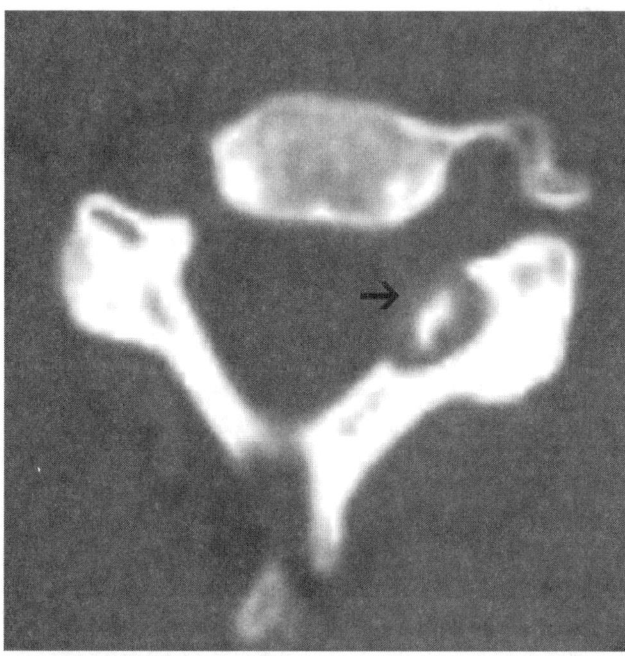

Axial CT of the C4 vertebrae with a sclerotic nidus at the laminar-pedicle junction (arrow) characteristic of an osteoid osteoma. (Adapted from Fast A, Goldsher D. *Navigating the Adult Spine: Bridging Clinical Practice and Neuroradiology*. New York: Demos Medical Publishing, 2007:113.)

### *Testing*

- X-rays can diagnose osteoid osteoma based on the characteristic surrounding area of dense sclerotic bone enclosing a radiolucent center that is 1.5 cm in diameter.
- May be difficult to detect on X-rays
- Bone scan demonstrates regions of tumor with increased activity.
- X-rays may also be used to monitor for local tumor recurrence.
- CT is used to determine the extent of bony involvement.
- CT-guided percutaneous biopsy may be used to resect accessible lesions.
- MRI is not routinely used.

### *Pitfalls*

- Several years may pass before a diagnosis is made.
- In skeletally immature patients, scoliosis may result in permanent scoliosis.
- Skeletally mature patients may have resolution of their scoliosis with surgical excision of the tumor.

## Red Flags

- Low back pain that worsens at night and is improved with aspirin in a young healthy adult may be mislabeled as psychogenic or malingering.
- Rare radicular symptoms

## Treatment

### *Medical*

- NSAIDs may be used for symptom control.

### *Exercises*

- None

### *Modalities*

- None

### *Injection*

- None

### *Surgical*

- Excision of the nidus and surrounding sclerotic bone may result in pain relief.
- Radiofrequency abalation may also be used to resolve the clinical symptoms.

### *Consults*

- Neurologic or orthopedic-spine surgery

### *Complications of treatment*

- Complications related to surgery

## Prognosis

- Recurrence is possible with incomplete excisions up to 10 years.
- Spontaneous resolution has been reported in the literature.
- No known cases of malignant transformation have been reported.

## Helpful Hints

- Full resection of the tumor can correct preoperative scoliosis and associated paraspinal muscle spasm.

## Suggested Readings

Kan P, Schmidt MH. Osteoid osteoma and osteoblastoma of the spine. *Neurosurg Clin N Am.* 2008;19(1):65–70.

Lee EH, Shafi M, Hui JH. Osteoid osteoma: a current review. *J Pediatr Orthop.* 2006;26(5):695–700.

# Osteomyelitis, Vertebral Body

## Description

Vertebral osteomyelitis refers to the growth of organisms within the bony structures of the axial spine.

## Etiology/Types

- Common organisms include *Staphylococcus aureus, Escherichia coli, Brucella abortus, Mycobacterium tuberculosis, Coccidiodes immitis, Treponema pallidum*, and *Echinococcus granulosus.*

## Epidemiology

- Incidence is estimated at 1 in 250,000.
- Up to 4% of all cases of osteomyelitis involve the vertebral body.
- The mean age is 45 to 62 years.
- The lumbar spine is the most commonly affected site followed by the thoracic spine, cervical spine, and sacrum.

## Pathogenesis

- Usually the result of hematogenous spread through Batson's plexus.
- May also occur through direct inoculation from interventional or surgical procedures.
- Vertebral body infection may spread into the adjacent soft tissue.
- The most common organism is *Staphylococcus aureus.*

## Risk Factors

- Alcoholism
- Chronic disease such as renal failure, HIV, and malignancy
- Dental extraction
- Genitourinary tract infection
- Infective endocarditis
- Intravenous drug use (*Pseudomonas aeruginosa*)
- Soft tissue infection
- Surgery: 1% for discectomy, and 6% for instrumented fusion

## Clinical Features

- Bacterial infections result in acute toxic reactions.
- Fungal or tuberculous infections are indolent reactions.

## Natural History

- Generally the pain develops over 8 to 12 weeks before the diagnosis is made.
- Progression of the infection may involve the surrounding soft tissues.

## Diagnosis

### *Differential diagnosis*

- Discitis
- Metastatic tumors
- Multiple myeloma
- Sarcoidosis

### *History*

- History of a recent interventional procedure or surgery
- Spinal pain corresponding to the level of involvement
- Constant or intermittent pain
- Pain improves with rest and worsens with motion.
- 30% may demonstrate radicular symptoms.
- Sore throat or dysphagia may occur with cervical involvement.

### *Exam*

- Fever
- Decreased spinal range of motion
- Tenderness over the involved spinal segment
- A psoas abscess may present with a hip flexor "contracture."
- Cervical presentation may include Horner's syndrome and torticollis.
- Possible neurologic deficits

### *Testing*

- During the acute phase, the white blood cell count and the erythrocyte sedimentation rate may be elevated
- The most useful test is direct culture of the blood and bony lesion.
- X-ray changes are delayed up to 2 months.
- Characteristic changes on X-rays include loss of vertebral body definition, bone loss, and narrowing of the disc space.
- Bone scan is positive earlier, within 72 hours after the onset of infection.
- SPECT may allow clearer visualization of infection within the posterior elements.
- CT demonstrates bony changes and penetration into the soft tissues

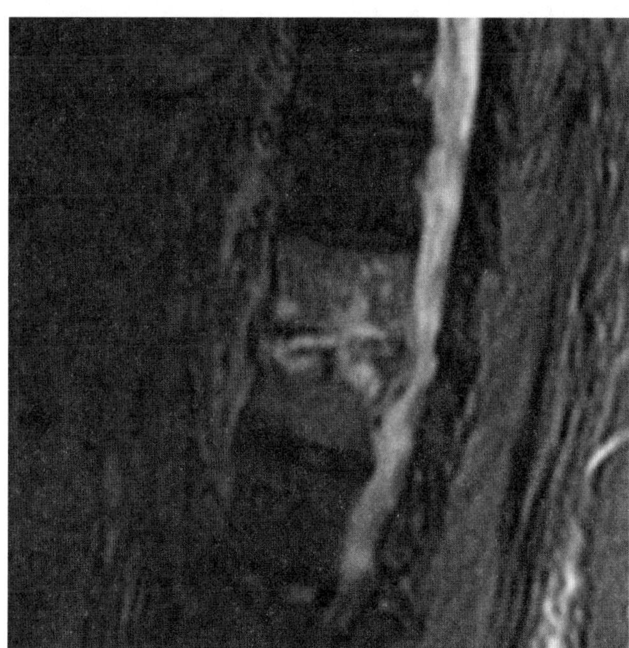

Sagittal thoracic T2-weighted magnetic resonance image with fat suppression demonstrates osteomyelitis of adjacent vertebral bodies with complete destruction of the intervertebral disc. (Courtesy of Keith Hentel, MD.)

- MRI is very sensitive in demonstrating the inflammatory process within the bony structure and surrounding soft tissue structures.

### *Pitfalls*

- Delayed diagnosis

## Red Flags

- Progressive spinal instability
- Progressive neurologic compromise

## Treatment

### *Medical*

- Antibiotic choice is governed by the culture results and may require up to 6 weeks of treatment followed by an oral course as long as 6 months, depending on the organism.
- Immobilization
- Bed rest

### *Exercises*

- None

### *Modalities*

- Modalities are contraindicated as they may increase the spread of the infectious process.

### *Injection*

- None

### *Surgical*

- Decompression and fusion may be required for patients who develop spinal instability.

### *Consults*

- Infectious disease
- Neurologic or orthopedic-spine surgery

### *Complications of treatment*

- Bony destruction may cause spinal instability.
- Spinal cord injury
- Complications related to delay in diagnosis, antibiotics, or surgical treatment

## Prognosis

- With early diagnosis and treatment, the patient will have minimal disability.
- Up to 10% of patients have a relapse with inadequate treatment.

## Helpful Hints

- Diagnosis is often missed.
- Mycobacterial osteomyelitis may take up to 3 years before a diagnosis is made.

## Suggested Reading

Concia E, Prandini N, Massari L, et al. Osteomyelitis: clinical update for practical guidelines. *Nucl Med Commun.* 2006;27(8):645–660.

# Osteoporosis

## Description

Osteoporosis is characterized by increased bone fragility and fractures resulting in increased morbidity and mortality.

## Etiology/Types

- Deterioration of the bone matrix leading to bone fragility

## Epidemiology

- 20% of white postmenopausal women in the United States have osteoporosis.
- One out of every two white women will experience an osteoporotic fracture at some point in her lifetime.
- The incidence of osteoporosis is lower in men due to larger bone mass and size, shorter lifespan, and the lack of a male menopausal state.

## Pathogenesis

- Caused by decreased estradiol after menopause in females and age-related bone metabolism changes as well as increased osteoclastic bone resorption, endocortical thinning, and an increasingly porous cortex

## Risk Factors

- Chronic obstructive pulmonary disease
- Eating disorders
- Female gender/athletic triad
- Gastrectomy
- Hyperparathyroidism
- Increasing age
- Low bone-mineral density
- Low body weight (<127 lbs)
- Malabsorption syndromes
- Greater number of deliveries and children breastfed

## Clinical Features

- Normal activities of daily living may result in a fracture in patients with severe osteoporosis.

## Natural History

- Impaired mobility and activities of daily living following a fracture

## Diagnosis

### *Differential diagnosis*

- Neoplasm

### *History*

- Inciting event
- Pain is improved with supine positioning.
- Worsens with walking or sitting

### *Exam*

- Bony tenderness at the fracture site
- Associated paraspinal muscle spasm
- Step-off deformity of the spinous processes
- Myelopathy due to retropulsion of the bony fragments into the central spinal canal
- Asymmetric leg positioning while supine
- Asymptomatic vertebral body compression fractures suspected with loss of >1.5 inches in serial height measurements or if the ribs touch the iliac crests

### *Testing*

- Urine calcium, serum thyrotropin, protein electrophoresis, cortisol, or anti-gliadin IgA and IgG antibodies to assess for celiac disease
- Older patients should be assessed for osteomalacia with a check of the 25-hydroxyvitamin D level.

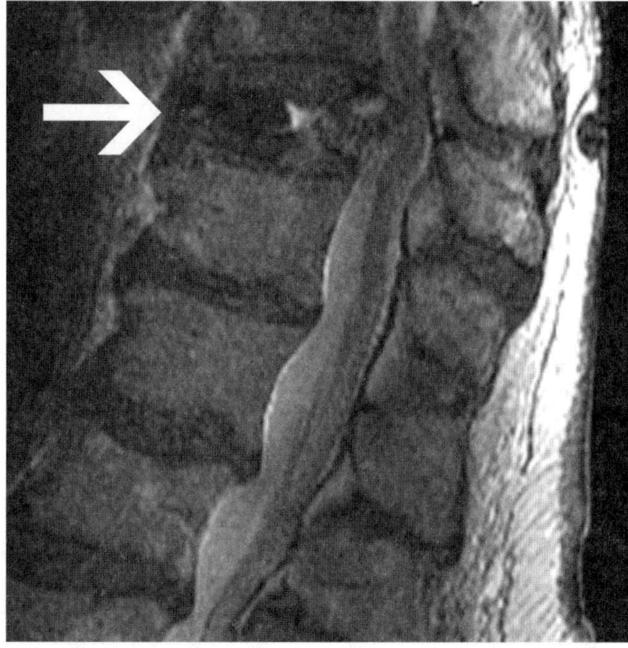

Sagittal lumbar T2-weighted magnetic resonance image demonstrating an osteoporotic T11 compression fracture with retropulsion of the posterior vertebral body wall into the central spinal canal.

- DEXA testing should start for women ≥65 years of age. In those at higher risk, testing should begin at 60 years of age.
- In males, testing should start at ≥70 years of age.
- Z score is the expected bone mineral density for the patient's age and sex.
- T score compares to "young, normal" adults of the same sex.
- Difference between the patient's score and the norm is expressed in standard deviations (SD) above or below the mean, where one SD equals 10% to 20% of the bone density value.
- Osteoporosis is defined as a bone mass density of ≥2.5 SD (T score ≤2.5) below the expected young adult mean bone mass density.
- 4.4-fold increase in future vertebral body fractures once a vertebral body fracture has occurred.

### *Pitfalls*

- Rule out other diseases that may have specific therapies available for treatment

## Red Flags

- Myelopathy

## Treatment

### *Medical*

- Therapy should be started in women when 1 of the following 3 criteria is met:
  - Bone mineral density T scores are below −2.0 with no risk factors,
  - Bone mineral density T scores below −1.5, with one or more risk factors
  - Prior vertebral or hip fracture
- Calcium and vitamin D
- Bisphosphonates
- Calcitonin
- Parathyroid hormone
- Selective estrogen receptor modulator
- Bracing

### *Exercises*

- Weight-bearing and strengthening exercises to improve balance and endurance
- Avoidance of flexion-based exercises

### *Modalities*

- Heat, cold, ultrasound, and transcutaneous electrical nerve stimulation have been used for symptomatic relief of pain and muscle spasms.

### *Injection*

- Percutaneous vertebral augmentation for acute or painful vertebral body fractures

### *Surgical*

- Fixation for unstable spine

### *Consults*

- Physical medicine and rehabilitation
- Neurologic or orthopedic-spine surgery
- Endocrinology

### *Complications of treatment*

- Continued pain
- Complications related to injection or surgery

## Prognosis

- Only 40% of hip fracture patients fully regain their prior level of independence.

## Helpful Hints

- Osteoporosis is undertreated because of inadequate screening and treatment.

## Suggested Readings

Bonnick SL. Osteoporosis in men and women. *Clin Cornerstone.* 2006;8(1):28–39.

Sinaki M. Exercise and osteoporosis. *Arch Phys Med Rehabil.* 1989;70(3):220–229.

# Paget's Disease

## Description

Paget's disease is a disorder characterized by localized bone resorption that is replaced by irregular new bone.

## Etiology/Types

- Unknown

## Epidemiology

- Affects up to 3% of individuals past the age of 40 and up to 10% of individuals 80 years of age
- Male to female ratio is 1.3:1

## Pathogenesis

- Primarily an abnormality of increased osteoclastic activity
- Osteoblastic activity
- Paramyxovirus infection
- Genetic predisposition

## Risk Factors

- Seven times increased risk of Paget's disease in first-degree relatives

## Clinical Features

- Most patients are asymptomatic.
- Most likely diagnosed due to increase alkaline phosphatase level or bony changes on radiographs.
- 43% of patients report back pain.
- Most often involves the sacrum, lumbar, thoracic, and cervical spines, in descending order.
- Bony changes may result in vertebral body fractures and nerve root compression.
- Cauda equina syndrome due to a spontaneous epidural hematoma
- May also affect the skull, femur, tibia, and pelvis resulting in increased skull size, hip joint osteoarthritis, and bowing of the legs.

## Natural History

- Most patients remain asymptomatic.

## Diagnosis

### *Differential diagnosis*

- Fibrous dysplasia
- Lymphoma
- Metastasis or neoplasm

### *History*

- Deep aching pain
- Pain worsened with weight-bearing
- No change with anti-inflammatory medications or rest
- Possible radicular component
- Classically associated with a change in hat size

### *Exam*

- May be normal
- Increased skull circumference
- Resting tachycardia
- Changes related to spinal cord injury
- Dorsal kyphosis with gait abnormality
- Bowing of the lower extremities
- Point tenderness over the involved spinal segments
- Scoliosis

### *Testing*

- Elevated alkaline phosphatase
- Hypercalcemia

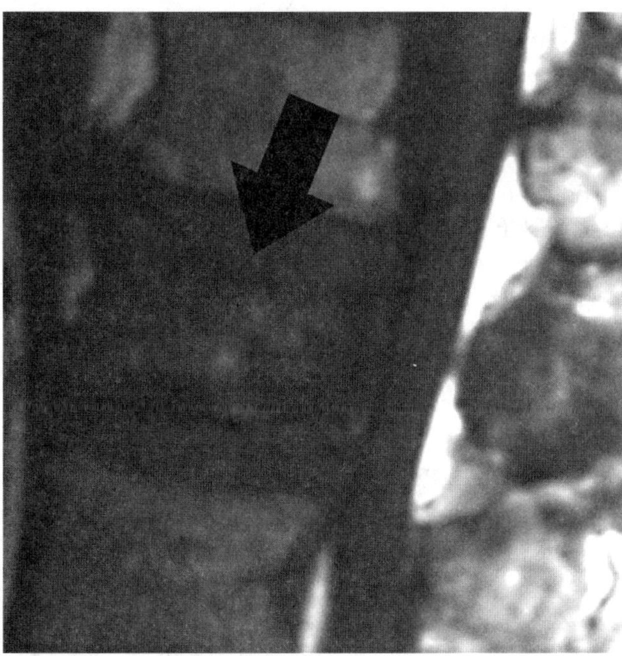

Sagittal T1-weighted magnetic resonance image demonstrating a hypointense vertebral body caused by bony sclerosis (arrow) compared with normal signal in the adjacent vertebral bodies. (Adapted from Fast A, Goldsher D. *Navigating the Adult Spine: Bridging Clinical Practice and Neuroradiology*. New York: Demos Medical Publishing, 2007:121.)

- Pathologically, the new bone formation resembles a mosaic pattern with normal material density.
- Plain radiographs may demonstrate lytic lesions in the skull, and rarely in the axial spine.
- Vertebral bodies may become enlarged.
- Bone scan can detect increased bony activity.
- CT demonstrates thickened trabeculae, although it is not required for diagnosis.

### *Pitfalls*

- Delayed diagnosis

## Red Flags

- Spinal cord injury
- Cauda equina syndrome

## Treatment

### *Medical*

- Calcitonin slows osteoclastic activity.
- Bisphosphonates decrease the ability of the osteoclasts to resorb bone.
- Mithramycin is cytotoxic agent used against osteoclasts.
- Screening should be performed every 4 to 6 months following remission

### *Exercises*

- General conditioning exercises to prevent deconditioning

### *Modalities*

- None

### *Injection*

- None

### *Surgical*

- Treatment required only for spinal decompression or weight-bearing joint replacement.

### *Consults*

- Rheumatology
- Neurologic or orthopedic surgery

### *Complications of treatment*

- Spinal cord injury
- Hypercalcemia with immobilization

## Prognosis

- Although there is no cure, most patients remain asymptomatic and require no therapy.
- The majority of patients achieve remission for at least 1 year.
- Malignant changes include malignant giant cell tumor, osteosarcoma, or fibrosarcoma.

## Helpful Hints

- Alkaline phosphatase levels should be followed every 4 to 6 months.

## Suggested Readings

Hadjipavlou AG, Gaitanis LN, Katonis PG, Lander P. Paget's disease of the spine and its management. *Eur Spine J.* 2001;10(5):370–384.

Whyte MP. Clinical practice. Paget's disease of bone. *N Engl J Med.* 2006;355(6):593–600.

# Psoriatic Arthritis

## Description

Psoriatic arthritis is a clinical syndrome of psoriasis of the skin or nails with a peripheral or axial inflammatory arthritis in the absence of a positive rheumatoid factor titer.

## Etiology/Types

- Unknown

## Epidemiology

- Estimated prevalence is 1% to 3% of the population
- Occurs in 5% to 7% of patients with psoriasis
- More common in populations in temperate climates
- No gender preference

## Pathogenesis

- Generally unknown, possibly related to metabolic abnormalities, bacterial infection, a delayed hypersensitivity inflammatory reaction, or trauma
- Synovial joints may be more susceptible to damage due to increased production of tumor necrosis factor-α, interleukin-1β, interleukin-2, and interleukin-10, and decreased production of interleukin-4 and -5.

## Risk Factors

- There is a family history in one-third of patients.
- HLA-B27 is more common with patients with axial spine disease.
- Susceptibility is thought to be based on chromosome 6.

## Clinical Features

- Variable clinical presentation with either arthritic or skin manifestations
- Most commonly associated with asymmetric oligoarthritis
- Patients <20 years of age may present with arthritis mutilans characterized by joint destruction.
- Dactylitis or diffuse swelling of the digit
- Axial spine disease typically occurs in males with later onset
- Morning stiffness
- Fatigue

## Natural History

- Unpredictable

## Diagnosis

### Differential diagnosis

- Gout
- Reactive arthritis
- Rheumatoid arthritis

### History

- Asymmetric oligoarthritis
- Fatigue
- Morning stiffness
- 80% of patients demonstrate pitting, horizontal ridging, and discoloration of nails.
- Skin plaques may be present.

### Exam

- Psoriatic skin plaques that appear as raised erythematous dry scaling lesions, most commonly over the scalp, elbows, and knees
- Skin plaques may be found in axial folds and the umbilicus.
- Nail bed changes
- Distal extremity swelling
- Pitting edema
- Loss of axial spine range of motion
- Unilateral or bilateral sacroiliac joint involvement

### Testing

- Rheumatoid factor and antinuclear antibodies are absent.
- Leukocytosis, anemia, and an elevated erythrocyte sedimentation rate
- Psoriatic joint fluid is unremarkable.
- X-rays may demonstrate a characteristic pencil-in-cup deformity with erosive changes in the distal interphalangeal joint and terminal phalanx.
  - Sacroiliitis demonstrates sclerosis and erosions within the ilium associated with joint widening.
  - Spondylitis is demonstrated with asymmetrical changes in the vertebral bodies and syndesmophytes.
- Bone scan may demonstrate increased activity before changes are noted on X-rays.
- CT and MRI may be used to assess unassociated neurologic deficits.

### Pitfalls

- The diagnosis may be missed if the clinician does not search for hidden psoriatic lesions.

## Red Flags

- Unassociated neurologic symptoms such as myelopathy or radiculopathy

## Treatment

### Medical

- Improved skin care correlates with changes in the arthritic component.
  - Skin care options include emollients, corticosteroids, tar shampoos, retinoids, and phototherapy.
- NSAIDs for joint pain and stiffness
- Corticosteroids are avoided due to the rebound effect following discontinuation
- Methotrexate
- Antitumor necrosis factor-α inhibitors

### Exercises

- General strengthening and stretching

### Modalities

- None

### Injection

- Corticosteroid joint injection

### Surgical

- None

### Consults

- Physical medicine and rehabilitation
- Rheumatology

### Complications of treatment

- Side effects related to medication management include liver toxicity with methotrexate and squamous cell skin cancer associated with retinoids.

## Prognosis

- 20% of patients develop joint destruction with significant disability.
- 97% of patients with psoriatic arthritis missed <12 months of work over a 10-year period.
- Increased severity of disease results in increased mortality.

## Helpful Hints

- Early treatment may result in better outcomes

## Suggested Readings

Gladman DD. Axial disease in psoriatic arthritis. *Curr Rheumatol Rep.* 2007;9(6):455–460.

Kleinert S, Feuchtenberger M, Kneitz C, Tony HP. Psoriatic arthritis: clinical spectrum and diagnostic procedures. *Clin Dermatol.* 2007;25(6):519–523.

# Radiculopathy, Cervical

## Description

Cervical radiculopathy is a pathological process involving compression and inflammation of a nerve root at the neuroforamen of the cervical spine.

## Etiology/Types

- Most commonly caused by a cervical disc herniation followed by spondylosis.
- Traumatic; caused by acute compression

## Epidemiology

- Annual incidence is 85 in 100,000.

## Pathogenesis

- Progressive loss of water from the disc (from 90% to 70%), leading to a more compressible and less elastic fibrocartilagenous mass.
- Disc bulges dorsally, the ligamentum flavum buckles ventrally, and the zygapophyseal (facet) joint capsules fold dorsally, resulting in narrowing of the central and foraminal canals.
- Reactive bone formation results in disc margin, uncovertebral, and zygapophyseal (facet) joint osteophytes.
- C7 root is the most commonly affected, followed in descending order by C6, C8, and C5.

## Risk Factors

- Genetic predisposition

## Clinical Features

- Neck pain associated with sharp radiating pain in the upper extremity along the affected nerve distribution
- Pain may interfere with work and sleep.
- Some patients may also present with weakness without significant pain or sensory changes

## Natural History

- Pain of an acute cervical radiculopathy may persist or diminish over time as the condition becomes chronic or resolves.

## Diagnosis

### *Differential diagnosis*

- Angina pectoris
- Cervical myelopathy
- Cervical spondylosis
- Intramedullary tumors
- Motor neuron disease
- Myocardial infarction
- Myofascial pain syndrome
- Peripheral nerve entrapment
- Plexopathy
- Shoulder pathology
- Syringomyelia
- Tendonitis
- Thoracic outlet disease

### *History*

- Neck pain with radiation down the arm
- Referred pain can be noted in the shoulder, interscapular, and suboccipital regions.

### *Exam*

- Motor weakness is the most reliable sign for localizing the affected nerve root.
- Decreased neck range of motion
- Spurling's test
- Shoulder abduction test relieves symptoms
- Axial manual distraction

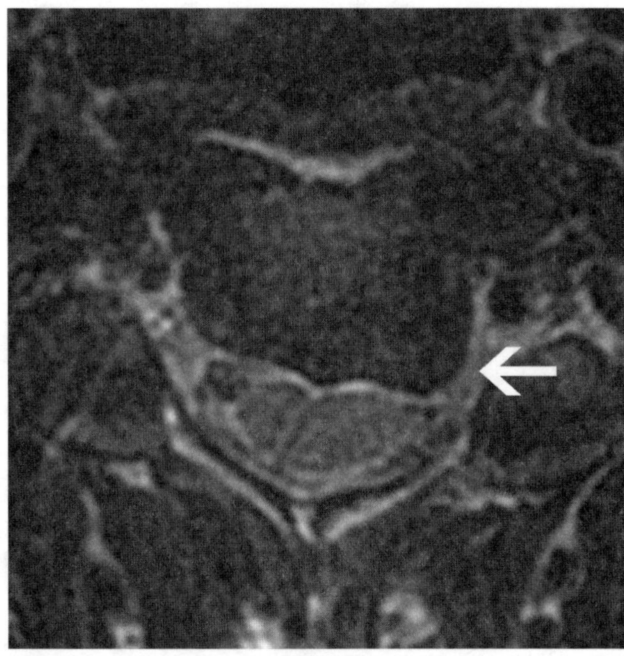

Axial cervical T2-weighted magnetic resonance image demonstrating a left lateral/ intraforaminal disc herniation (arrow).

### Testing
- X-rays are useful in trauma, deformity, instability, infection, inflammatory disease, or neoplasms.
- MRI is the best imaging study to evaluate nerve root pathology.
- Disc herniations may be found in 5% to 10% of asymptomatic people and disc degeneration is noted in 25% to 60% of asymptomatic individuals.
- CT scans can rule out fractures and add further bony delineation of the foraminal region.
- Electrodiagnostic studies can be useful in diagnosis and ruling out other neurologic conditions.

### Pitfalls
- Weakness greater than three-fifth is rare due to multiple innervations of the muscles of the upper extremity (except for the rhomboids).
- Sensory changes often do not match classical dermatomal distributions.
- Pin-prick and/or light-touch sensory evaluations should be done at the distal aspects of the dermatomes, as parasthesias and numbness are more common distally than motor loss or deep tendon reflex changes.
- The pronator reflex helps differentiate a C6 root from a C7 root lesion.
- May be difficult to differentiate C8 root involvement from an ulnar entrapment at the elbow.
- Caution should be used as disc herniations have also been found on MRI in 5% to 10% of asymptomatic individuals.

## Red Flags
- Myelopathy

## Treatment

### Medical
- NSAIDs
- Analgesics
- Anticonvulsants
- Muscle relaxants
- Oral corticosteroid taper

### Exercises
- Physical therapy focuses on stretching and strengthening exercises of the cervical paraspinal, shoulder, and upper back muscles.
- Ergonomic assessment focused on improved posture with the goal of neutral positioning.
- Traction

### Modalities
- Heat, cold, ultrasound, and transcutaneous electrical nerve stimulation have been used for symptomatic relief of pain and muscle spasms.

### Injection
- Trigger point injections for symptoms of myofascial pain
- Epidural steroid injection for radicular symptoms

### Surgical
- Surgery is considered for patients with severe intractable pain, significant weakness, or myelopathy impacting functional mobility.

### Consults
- Physical medicine and rehabilitation
- Neurologic or orthopedic-spine surgery

### Complications of treatment
- Development of chronic pain
- Complications related to epidural steroid injections

## Prognosis
- 80% to 90% of patients have good results with conservative management.

## Helpful Hints
- Cervical radiculopathy may go undiagnosed if it does not fit a classic pattern.

## Suggested Reading
Abbed KM, Coumans JVCE. Cervical radiculopathy: pathophysiology, presentation, and clinical evaluation. *Neurosurgery.* 2007;60(Suppl 1):S28–S34.

# Radiculopathy, Lumbar

## Description

Lumbar radiculopathy is a pathological process involving compression and inflammation of a nerve root at the neuroforamen of the lumbar spine.

## Etiology/Types

- Etiology includes mechanical overload, repetitive strain, or trauma.

## Epidemiology

- Most commonly in individuals 30 to 50 years of age, although it may occur in older individuals.

## Pathogenesis

- 90% of lesions occur at the L5–S1 followed by the L4–L5 intervertebral levels.
- Central herniations will impinge the nerve root exiting one level below, whereas a far lateral herniation will impinge the nerve root exiting at the same level.
- Larger disc herniations are resorbed more often than smaller herniations.
- Pain associated with a disc herniation is related to compression of the nerve root and/or the release of inflammatory mediators.

## Risk Factors

- Flexion with rotation
- Genetic predisposition

## Clinical Features

- Previous history of low back pain
- Lower back pain with radiation down the leg
- Positive straight leg raise associated with the loss of deep tendon reflexes, motor weakness, and numbness associated with a single nerve root.

## Natural History

- Disc herniation may be self-limiting, although it may be accompanied by pain and limited activities, which results in deconditioning.

## Diagnosis

### *Differential diagnosis*

- Hip joint pathology
- Sacroiliac joint dysfunction
- Spinal stenosis
- Spondylosis

### *History*

- Mild or severe sharp pain that can radiate down the leg along the distribution of the affected nerve.
- Patients may only have lower back pain with radiation into the buttocks.

### *Exam*

- Functional scoliosis
- Antalgic gait
- Decreased lumbar range of motion
- Positive straight leg raise
- Paraspinals and gluteus medius tenderness
- An L5 radiculopathy presents as weakness of the extensor hallucis longus muscle, loss of the ankle reflex, and decreased sensation at the web space between the first and second toes.
- An S1 radiculopathy presents as gastrocnemius-soleus weakness manifesting with the inability to toe walk or do 10 successive toe raises, loss of the ankle reflex, and sensory loss at the lateral malleolus and posterior calf.
- Presentation can be variable, often with no objective reflex, motor, or sensory findings.

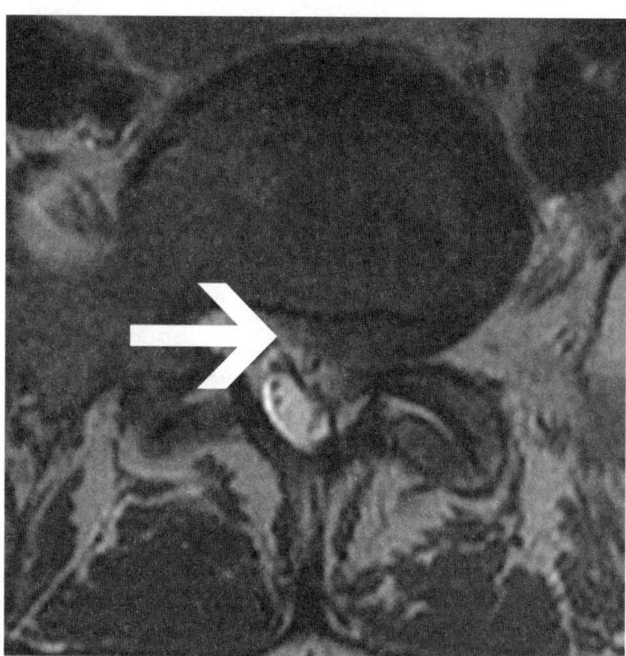

Axial lumbar T2-weighted magnetic resonance image demonstrating a large left L4–L5 paracentral disc herniation displacing the thecal sac.

### Testing

- Electrodiagnostic studies confirm nerve impingement and in some cases the chronicity of nerve root damage.
- CT may demonstrate a disc herniation.
- MRI allows for visualization of the disc herniation and the affected nerve root.

### Pitfalls

- Caution should be used as disc herniations have also been found on MRI in 20% to 57% of asymptomatic individuals.

## Red Flags

- Severe motor weakness
- Cauda equina syndrome

## Treatment

### Medical

- NSAIDs
- Analgesics
- Anticonvulsants
- Muscle relaxants
- Oral corticosteroid taper

### Exercises

- Bed rest is not recommended beyond 2 days, if at all.
- Walking should be encouraged.
- Gradual stretching and strengthening
- McKenzie extension-based positioning

### Modalities

- Heat, cold, ultrasound, and transcutaneous electrical nerve stimulation have been used for symptomatic relief of pain and muscle spasms.

### Injection

- Trigger point injections for symptoms of myofascial pain
- Epidural steroid injections can be used for symptomatic control to allow the patient to return to a pain-free state and progress in physical therapy.
- Transforaminal steroid injections have been shown to have a success rate of 84% compared to 48% of those receiving trigger point injections.
  - Benefits may last up to 16 months
  - Symptoms may also never recur

### Surgical

- Laminectomy or microdiscectomy for patients who have failed conservative treatment, or who demonstrate progressive neurologic deterioration or cauda equina syndrome.

### Consults

- Physical medicine and rehabilitation
- Neurologic surgery or orthopedic-spine surgery

### Complications of treatment

- Lasting neurologic deficit
- Chronic pain
- Complications related to epidural steroid injections

## Prognosis

- 80% of patients will respond to conservative treatment.
- Surgical discectomy has been found to be successful in young patients with 85% reporting decreased leg pain and 75% reporting decreased back pain.
- Recurrent disc herniations occur in 6% of patients.

## Helpful Hints

- MRI has not been found to be predictive of future symptoms related to disc herniation.

## Suggested Reading

Tarulli AW, Raynor EM. Lumbosacral radiculopathy. *Neurol Clin.* 2007;25(2):387–405.

# Radiculopathy, Thoracic

## Description

Thoracic radiculopathy is a pathological process involving compression and inflammation of a nerve root at the neuroforamen of the thoracic spine.

## Etiology/Types

- Most commonly due to disc degeneration

## Epidemiology

- 0.15% to 4% of all symptomatic disc herniations occur in the thoracic spine.
- Most common in the third to sixth decades of life

## Pathogenesis

- Thoracic central canal is small compared with cervical and lumbar canals, increasing risk of injury.
- The bony rib cage of the first 10 thoracic vertebral bodies limits flexion and rotation, protecting the thoracic spine.
- Increased risk at the lower thoracic levels due to increased motion
- All thoracic levels have been associated with a disc herniation.
- T8–T12 levels are the most commonly involved sites.
- 26% to 50% of all thoracic disc herniations occur at the T11–T12 level.
- Approximately 37% of thoracic disc herniations are asymptomatic.
- Typically posterocentral or posterolateral with rare lateral herniations
- Most thoracic disc protrusions occur centrally and directly compress or create traction on the spinal cord.

## Risk Factors

- Preexisting disc degeneration
- Scheuermann's disease
- Trauma

## Clinical Features

- Variable history of pain and dysesthesias across the affected nerve root innervating the chest, thorax, or abdomen
- Important landmarks are the nipple line at T4, the xyphoid process at T6, and the umbilicus at T10.
- Characteristic tenderness at the affected thoracic spine level
- Pain is the most common symptom followed by sensory changes, lower extremity motor changes and bladder symptoms.

## Natural History

- Progressive disc degeneration may worsen symptoms, which may lead to paraplegia.

## Diagnosis

### *Differential diagnosis*

- Angina pectoris
- Arteriovenous malformation
- Costochondritis
- Degenerative disc disease
- Diabetes mellitus–related radiculopathy
- Dyspepsia
- Herpes zoster
- Infection
- Intercostal neuralgia
- Osteomalacia
- Osteoporosis
- Peripheral neuropathy
- Primary or metastatic neoplasm
- Pulmonary or hepatobiliary causes
- Somatic dysfunction/myofascial pain
- Thoracic spinal stenosis (often associated with lumbar stenosis)
- Vertebral body or rib fracture

### *History*

- Burning aching sensation following a dermatomal pattern across chest, thorax, or abdomen
- Back, leg, or thoracic pain
- Gait disturbance

### *Exam*

- Unreliable
- Localized spine and paraspinal tenderness
- Sensory changes
- No isolated muscle testing available

### *Testing*

- MRI is the most sensitive test and is used to assess for other pathology.
- CT scan
- Electrodiagnostic studies should include needle EMG of the involved intercostal, abdominal, and thoracic paraspinal muscles.

- Used to rule out a polyneuropathy

### Pitfalls

- T1 radiculopathies primarily affect the ulnar aspect of the proximal arm.
- Months or years before the diagnosis is made
- Need to rule out myelopathy

## Red Flags

- Progressive myelopathy accompanying the presenting radiculopathy

## Treatment

### Medical

- Bed rest for <2 days, if at all
- NSAIDs
- Analgesics
- Anticonvulsants
- Muscle relaxants
- Oral corticosteroid taper

### Exercises

- General strengthening and stretching
- Trunk stabilization

### Modalities

- Heat, cold, ultrasound, and transcutaneous electrical nerve stimulation have been used for symptomatic relief of pain and muscle spasms.

### Injection

- Trigger point injections for symptoms of myofascial pain
- Epidural steroid injection for radicular symptoms
- Intercostal nerve blocks for intercostal neuralgia

### Surgical

- Indication includes "bandlike" chest pain, paraparesis.
- Posterior surgical laminectomy not preferred due to spinal cord injury resulting from excessive mobilization of the thoracic spinal cord to access the anterior disc herniation.
- Laminectomy is possible with far lateral herniations.
- Anterior approach for central disc herniations
- Video-assisted thoracoscopic surgery approaches are preferred.

### Consults

- Physical medicine and rehabilitation
- Neurologic or orthopedic-spine surgery

### Complications of treatment

- Paraparesis or paraplegia
- Complications related to epidural steroid injections

## Prognosis

- Up to 77% of patients treated conservatively have been able to return to their premorbid functional level.
- Diabetes mellitus–related radiculopathy has a self-limiting course of 6 to 18 months.

## Helpful Hints

- Underdiagnosed condition

## Suggested Reading

O'Connor RC, Andary MT, Russo RB, DeLano M. Thoracic radiculopathy. *Phys Med Rehabil Clin N Am.* 2002;13(3):623.

# Rheumatoid Arthritis

## Description

Rheumatoid arthritis (RA) is a chronic, systemic, inflammatory, immune-mediated disease of the synovial joints.

## Etiology/Types

- Probably associated with genetic (HLA-DR1 and HLA-DR4) and environmental factors such as viral infection.

## Epidemiology

- Most commonly diagnosed in persons between the ages of 40 and 70 years
- 80% of patients demonstrate cervical spine manifestations.
- Up to 5% of RA patients have lumbar spine and sacroiliac joint involvement.
- 7% to 10% of RA patients develop neurologic manifestations.

## Pathogenesis

- Proinflammatory cytokines (tumor necrosis factor-α and interleukin-1) lead to synovial inflammation, causing synovial membrane hypertrophy and joint destruction.

## Risk Factors

- Unknown genetic and environmental risk factors

## Clinical Features

- The American Rheumatism Association's 1987 classification criteria for rheumatoid arthritis recommends diagnosis if four of the following seven criteria are met:
  - Morning stiffness
  - Involvement of three or more joints
  - Hand joint involvement
  - Symmetrical arthritis
  - Rheumatoid nodules
  - Positive rheumatoid factor
  - Documented radiographic changes
- Swollen and painful synovial joints of the cervical spine, hands, wrists, elbows, hips, knees, ankles, and feet
- Signs in the cervical spine include decreased range of motion and neurologic dysfunction such as parasthesias, bowel or bladder dysfunction, or tetraplegia.

## Natural History

- Affected cervical components include the atlas and axis, zygapophyseal (facet) and uncovertebral joints, and surrounding bursa.
- 25% of RA patients have erosion of the C1–C2 complex.
- 29% of patients may have subluxation at the C3–C4 and C4–C5 levels.
- Peripheral joint destruction

## Diagnosis

### *Differential diagnosis*

- Ankylosing spondylitis
- Local infection
- Psoriatic arthritis
- Reactive arthritis

### *History*

- Characteristic joint pain, tenderness, swelling, and erythema most likely present at the proximal interphalangeal and carpometacarpal joints as well as the wrist, elbows, hip, knee, ankle, and metatarsophalangeal joints.
- Worsens in the morning or with inactivity and improves with activity
- Cervical subluxation may develop with little peripheral involvement
- Lumbar-pain severity is associated with the severity of the peripheral disease
- Mild sacroiliac joint pain

### *Exam*

- Peripheral joint manifestations include erythematous, tender and boggy joints, and loss of range of motion.
- Neck and lumbar range of motion may be diminished with associated bony or paraspinal tenderness.
- Upper-extremity weakness, numbness, or tingling
- Myelopathy

### *Testing*

- Positive rheumatoid factor, elevated erythrocyte sedimentation rate, anemia, and thrombocytosis
- Synovial fluid is characteristic of inflammatory fluid.
- X-rays of the extremities demonstrate soft tissue swelling, joint space narrowing, bony erosion, and periarticular osteopenia.

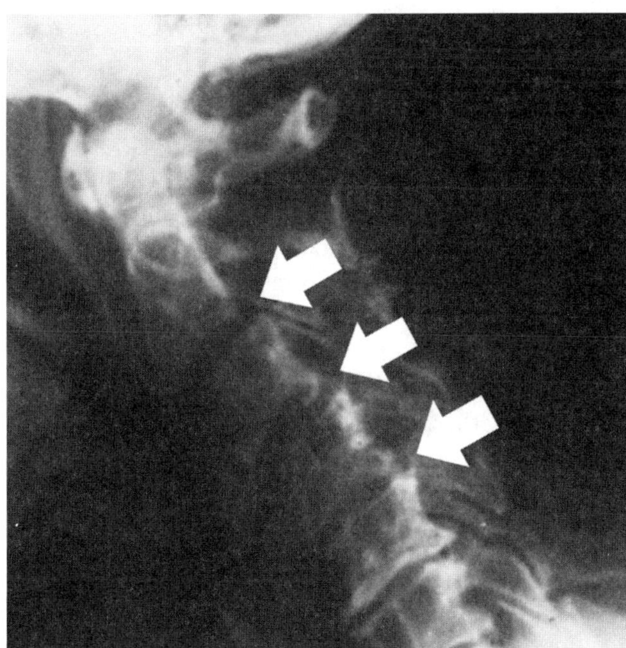

Lateral cervical plain radiograph demonstrating subaxial instability (arrows) due to facet joint destruction and ligament laxity found in rheumatoid arthritis. (Adapted from Fast A, Goldsher D. *Navigating the Adult Spine: Bridging Clinical Practice and Neuroradiology*. New York: Demos Medical Publishing, 2007:90.)

- Cervical spine X-rays should include open-mouth odontoid views.
- CT is used to determine bony destruction.
- MRI is useful in determining the extent of soft tissue disruption as well as spinal cord injury.

### *Pitfalls*
- Overlooked cervical subluxation

## Red Flags
- Paresthesias
- Dysphagia/dysarthria
- Myelopathy
- Subluxation with vertebral artery compression may result in tetraplegia, coma, or death.

## Treatment

### *Medical*
- NSAIDs
- Disease-modifying antirheumatic drugs
- Corticosteroids
- Antitumor necrosis factor-α inhibitors
- Rigid collars can limit anterior subluxation but are not generally tolerated.

### *Exercises*
- Gentle strengthening and stretching exercises

### *Modalities*
- Heat, cold, ultrasound, and transcutaneous electrical nerve stimulation have been used for symptomatic relief of pain and muscle spasms.

### *Injection*
- None

### *Surgical*
- Spinal stabilization may be required in patients with progressive neurologic deficits, although the fusion rate is only 50%.

### *Consults*
- Rheumatology
- Physical medicine and rehabilitation
- Neurologic or orthopedic-spine surgery

### *Complications of treatment*
- 10% mortality associated with surgery

## Prognosis
- RA patients with subluxation have an eightfold higher mortality compared to those with RA alone.

## Helpful Hints
- Early diagnosis and treatment minimizes later functional deficits

## Suggested Reading
Oh TH, Lim PA, Brander VA, Kaelin DL. Rehabilitation of orthopedic and rheumatologic disorders. 2. Connective tissue diseases. *Arch Phys Med Rehabil.* 2000;81(3 Suppl 1):S60–S66.

# Sacroiliac Joint Pain

## Description
Pain originating from the sacroiliac joint

## Etiology/Types
- Enthesopathy
- Fracture
- Myofascial pain
- Ligamentous injury
- Arthritis
- Infection

## Epidemiology
- Thought to be the cause of 15% to 30% of chronic low back pain cases.
- Up to 32% of patients with lumbosacral spinal fusion develop sacroiliac joint pain.

## Pathogenesis
- The sacroiliac joint allows vertical forces to be transferred between the lower extremities and the trunk.
- Diarthodial joint lined with hyaline cartilage with two irregular bony surfaces formed by the sacrum and ilium
- The superior third of the joint is attached to the surrounding ligaments.
- The joint surface of the inferior third of the sacroiliac joint is similar to a synovial joint.
- Unique, as there are no muscles that act on the joint.
- Only 2 to 3 degrees of joint motion
- Thought to be innervated posteriorly by the lateral branches of the L4–S1 posterior rami and anteriorly from the L2–S2 segments.

## Risk Factors
- Altered posture
- Athletes involved in unilateral lower-extremity loading, such as throwing or kicking
- Cross-country skiers
- Increased lordosis
- Pregnancy-related weight gain, increased lordotic posture, parturition, and the release of relaxin
- Trauma
- Weight gain

## Clinical Features
- May present with low back pain, pelvic pain, sacral pain, or gluteal pain
- Variable somatic referred-pain patterns, which include the buttocks, lumbar region, lower extremity, groin, abdomen, lower leg, and foot
- Unilateral pain is four times more common than bilateral pain.

## Natural History
- With aging there is no fusion, but there is increased stiffness and joint-space narrowing.

## Diagnosis

### *Differential diagnosis*
- Ankylosing spondylitis
- Discogenic pain
- Hip joint pathology
- Malignancy
- Myofascial pain
- Radiculopathy
- Referred visceral pain
- Rheumatoid arthritis
- Trochanteric bursitis
- Zygapophyseal (facet) joint pain

### *History*
- Numbness, clicking, popping, or groin pain
- Unilateral or bilateral buttock pain
- Pain below or medial to the posterior superior iliac spine
- Pain increases when arising from a sitting position or with bending or twisting

### *Exam*
- Likelihood of diagnosing sacroiliac joint pain is increased if three or more provocative tests are positive.
  - Flexion abduction external rotation (FABER) test
  - Distraction/compression test
  - Focal sacroiliac joint tenderness
  - Gillet's test
  - Modified Gaenslen's test

### *Testing*
- X-rays and MRI can be used to assess for sacral fractures, ankylosing spondylitis, sacroiliitis, and tumors.
- Image-guided contrast-enhanced sacroiliac joint injection

### *Pitfalls*
- Misdiagnosis

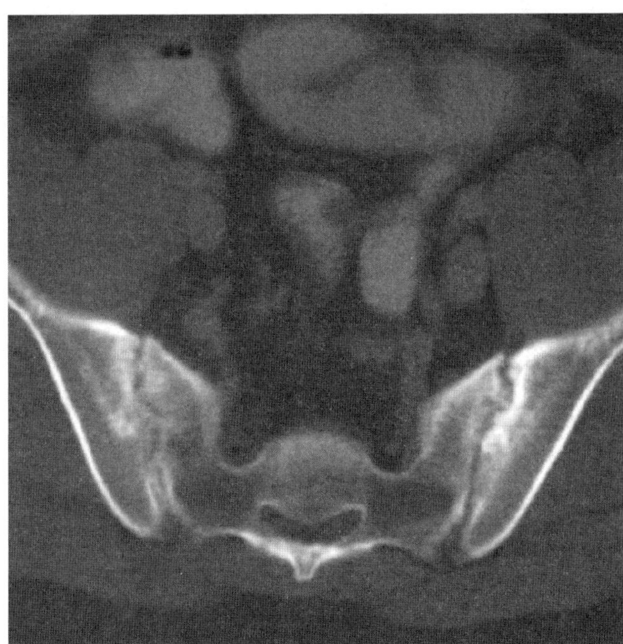

Axial computed tomography scan of the sacroiliac joints demonstrates bilateral sclerotic changes and joint-space narrowing.

## Red Flags

- Infection
- Tumor

## Treatment

### Medical

- Relative rest for acute injuries
- NSAIDs
- Analgesics
- Sacroiliac joint belt, especially in pregnancy-related pain

### Exercises

- Focus on correcting strength and muscle imbalance
- Pelvic girdle muscle strengthening
- Joint mobilization
- Muscle energy techniques

### Modalities

- Heat, cold, ultrasound, and transcutaneous electrical nerve stimulation have been used for symptomatic relief of pain and muscle spasms.

### Injection

- Fluoroscopically guided contrast-enhanced sacroiliac joint injection
- Ultrasound-guided sacroiliac joint injections
- Blind injections have been found to penetrate the joint in only 22% of attempts.
- Radiofrequency neurotomy

### Surgical

- Surgery is reserved for infections, displaced fractures, or instability.

### Consults

- Physical medicine and rehabilitation
- Orthopedic-spine surgery

### Complications of treatment

- Fluoroscopically guided contrast-enhanced sacroiliac joint injection may block the sacral plexus anteriorly or the L5 and S1 nerve roots, resulting in weakness or numbness.

## Prognosis

- Good with a definitive diagnosis

## Helpful Hints

- Always consider the sacroiliac joint in patients with low back pain.

## Suggested Reading

Foley BS, Buschbacher RM. Sacroiliac joint pain: anatomy, biomechanics, diagnosis, and treatment. *Am J Phys Med Rehabil.* 2006;85(12):997–1006.

# Sarcoidosis

## Description

Sarcoidosis is a disease that results in the formation of inflammatory granulomas primarily in the lung and thoracic lymph nodes with occasional involvement of the thoracolumbar spine.

## Etiology/Types

- Unknown

## Epidemiology

- Prevalence of 1 per 10,000
- More common in African Americans
- Age of onset ranges between 20 and 40 years of age
- No gender preference

## Pathogenesis

- Though to be caused by immune dysfunction resulting from unknown genetic and environmental factors
- Characterized by delayed hypersensitivity, CD4/CD8 T cell imbalance, B cell hyperactivity, accumulation of Th1 helper cells at the site of activity, and circulating immune complexes
- Inflammatory granulomas develop anywhere in the body, although are most commonly found in the lung and adjacent thoracic lymph nodes.
- Inflammatory granulomas cause tissue fibrosis resulting in organ dysfunction or failure.
- Bony involvement is less common but can affect the skull, ribs, humerus, femur, ribs, hands, and feet.
- Rare involvement of the vertebral bodies, sacroiliac, and hip joints

## Risk Factors

- Unknown

## Clinical Features

- Cough
- Shortness of breath
- Pain at the site of vertebral involvement
- Osseous involvement generally occurs in local proximity to the clinical or radiographic pulmonary involvement, which correlates to the lower thoracic and upper lumbar levels.
- Pathologic fracture is possible.

## Natural History

- Progressive granuloma formation may lead to vertebral body collapse.

## Diagnosis

### *Differential diagnosis*

- Hodgkin's lymphoma
- Metastasis
- Osteomyelitis
- Tuberculosis

### *History*

- Fever
- Weight loss
- Dull stabbing pain at the involved spinal segment
- Pain worsened with activity and improved with rest
- Neurologic symptoms related to spinal cord compression, including bowel or bladder dysfunction
- Radicular symptoms

### *Exam*

- Point tenderness to palpation of the involved spinal segment
- Motor, sensory, and reflex changes in the lower extremities
- Ocular inflammation
- Skin rash
- Lymphadenopathy
- Abnormal pulmonary examination
- Splenomegaly

### *Testing*

- Laboratory findings may include increased alkaline phosphatase, hypercalcemia, hypergammaglobulinemia, elevated angiotensin-converting enzyme.
- Loss of delayed hypersensitivity inflammatory reaction
- Histologic confirmation of noncaseating granulomas
- X-rays demonstrate bony lysis with marginal sclerosis in the vertebral body with occasional disease activity in the posterior elements, which looks similar to metastatic disease.
- Electrocardiogram
- Ophthalmologic evaluation
- Bone scan demonstrates increased uptake at sites of active inflammation and is used to screen for extrathoracic granulomas.

- CT and MRI can be used to assess for neurosarcoidosis.

### *Pitfalls*

- Bony sarcoidosis has a similar appearance on X-rays to metastatic disease and intervertebral disc involvement may look like disciitis.

## Red Flags

- Signs of spinal cord compression
- Progressive radiculopathy
- Fracture

## Treatment

### *Medical*

- Corticosteroids over 6 to 12 months to decrease the inflammatory component
- Methotrexate may take up to 6 months to demonstrate effectiveness.

### *Exercises*

- Gentle strengthening and stretching

### *Modalities*

- None

### *Injection*

- None

### *Surgical*

- Biopsy may be required to confirm the diagnosis.
- Surgical decompression for spinal cord or nerve root compression
- Surgical fusion may be required for spinal instability.

### *Consults*

- Rheumatology
- Neurologic or orthopedic-spine surgery
- Cardiology
- Ophthalmology
- Other specialties based on organ involvement

### *Complications of treatment*

- Paraplegia
- Cauda equina syndrome
- Chronic radiculopathy
- Complications related to surgery

## Prognosis

- Good prognosis with vertebral involvement
- Generally extrathoracic involvement usually indicates more extensive systemic disease, which may correlate with a poorer prognosis.

## Helpful Hints

- Most sarcoid granulomas resolve, leaving little or no evidence of previous inflammation.

## Suggested Readings

Cohen NP, Gosset J, Staron RB, Levine WN. Vertebral sarcoidosis of the spine in a football player. *Am J Orthop.* 2001;30(12):875–877.

Mangino D, Stover DE. Sarcoidosis presenting as metastatic bony disease. A case report and review of the literature on vertebral body sarcoidosis. *Respiration.* 2004;71(3):292–294.

# Scheuermann's Disease

## Description

Scheuermann's disease is a progressive thoracic kyphosis.

## Etiology/Types

- Unknown

## Epidemiology

- Affects up to 8.3% of the general population.
- Primarily affects the thoracic spine, although it has also been noted in the lumbar spine.
- Most common in teenagers
- No gender preference

## Pathogenesis

- Caused by irregular ossification and endochondral growth at the junction of the intervertebral disc and vertebral body, resulting in wedging of the vertebral bodies and progressive kyphosis

## Risk Factors

- Genetic predisposition

## Clinical Features

- Up to 60% of individuals have back pain.
- Back pain at the location of the progressive scoliosis
- Decreased range of motion of the affected spinal segment
- Cardiopulmonary compromise may occur with a thoracic kyphosis >100 degrees, compared to a normal thoracic kyphosis measured from T5 to T12 that ranges from 20 to 40 degrees.

## Natural History

- Progressive scoliosis

## Diagnosis

### *Differential diagnosis*

- Hyperparathyroidism
- Neoplasm
- Paget's disease
- Rheumatoid arthritis
- Tuberculosis

### *History*

- Progressive kyphosis with associated back pain
- Pain improved with bed rest and worsened with activity.

### *Exam*

- Sharply angled kyphotic deformity most common in the thoracic region
- Kyphotic deformity may also be found in the thoracolumbar or lumbar region.
- Increased compensatory cervical and lumbar lordosis
- Kyphosis does not reduce with extension.
- Paravertebral muscle spasm or tension
- Scoliosis may also be present.

### *Testing*

- X-rays demonstrate vertebral body wedging, irregular endplates with penetrating Schmorl's nodes, and kyphosis.
- A minimum of three adjacent vertebrae wedged at least 5 degrees is used as a radiographic diagnostic criteria.

### *Pitfalls*

- Overlooking cardiopulmonary deficits

## Red Flags

- Spinal cord compression
- Thoracic disc herniation
- Cardiopulmonary compromise

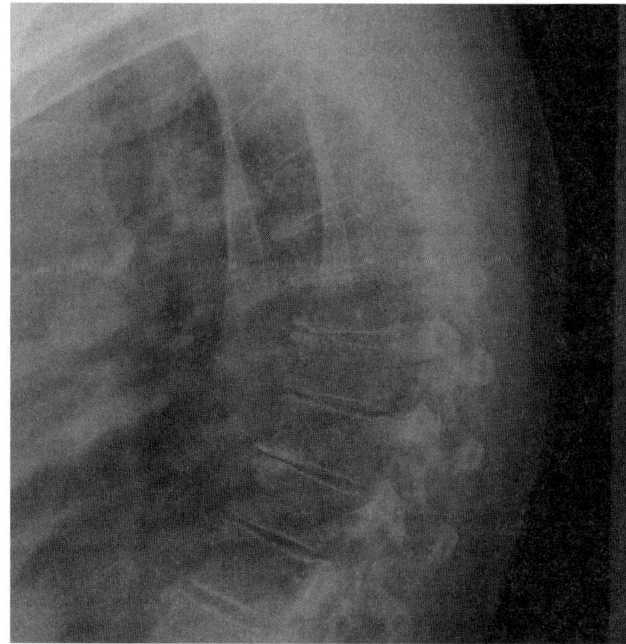

Lateral thoracic plain radiograph demonstrating wedging of the adjacent vertebrae, endplate irregularities, and a thoracic kyphosis of greater than 45 degrees, which is characteristic of Scheuermann's disease.

## Treatment

### Medical

- NSAIDs and analgesics for pain control
- Body casting or the use of a Milwaukee brace for progressive deformity
- The Milwaukee brace has been shown to prevent deformity in up to 40% of patients if used until skeletal maturity.

### Exercises

- Bed rest and back extensor muscle strengthening can be used to prevent progression in mild and reversible kyphosis.

### Modalities

- Heat, cold, ultrasound, and transcutaneous electrical nerve stimulation have been used for symptomatic relief of pain and muscle spasms.

### Injection

- Discography has been used to identify symptomatic levels.

### Surgical

- Operative management is considered in adolescents with >70 degrees of kyphosis.
- Operative management is considered in adults with progressive pain and deformity or progressive neurologic and cardiopulmonary deficits with a kyphosis of >100 degrees.

### Consults

- Physical medicine and rehabilitation
- Neurologic or orthopedic-spine surgery
- Pulmonology
- Cardiology

### Complications of treatment

- Spinal cord injury
- Cardiopulmonary compromise
- Complications related to surgery

## Prognosis

- Patients with kyphosis of >70 degrees may have continued progression after skeletal maturity.
- Continued kyphosis may result in continued back pain

## Helpful Hints

- In skeletally immature patients, it is important to follow the kyphotic progression.

## Suggested Readings

Kapetanos GA, Hantzidis PT, Anagnostidis KS, Kirkos JM. Thoracic cord compression caused by disk herniation in Scheuermann's disease: a case report and review of the literature. *Eur Spine J.* 2006;15(Suppl 5):553–558.

Lonner BS, Newton P, Betz R, et al. Operative management of Scheuermann's kyphosis in 78 patients: radiographic outcomes, complications, and technique. *Spine.* 2007;32(24):2644–2652.

# Schwannoma

## Description

A schwannoma is a solitary benign Schwann cell tumor that is found on sensory nerve roots.

## Etiology/Types

- Thought to arise from Schwann cells at the dorsal roots, the anterior spinal artery, or aberrant intramedullary nerve fibers

## Epidemiology

- Prevalence unknown
- Make up to 35% of all primary intraspinal tumors
- Occur in patients between 30 and 40 years of age
- 30% occur in the lumbar region.
- No gender preference
- More common in the cervical and lumbosacral regions

## Pathogenesis

- Commonly benign
- Encapsulated and typically round tumors that are attached to the nerve root.
- Vascular supply may originate from branches of the anterior spinal artery

## Risk Factors

- Unknown

## Clinical Features

- Neurologic dysfunction
- No pain initially, but pain usually develops
- Pain worsens with recumbent positioning
- Sensory or motor dysfunction related to a space-occupying lesion
- May occur in the cervical spine or sacrum
- May eventually erode the vertebral body, pedicles, or foramen

## Natural History

- Slow growing

## Diagnosis

### *Differential diagnosis*

- Herniated nucleus pulposus
- Meningioma
- Neurofibroma
- Spinal stenosis

### *History*

- Pain
- Motor and sensory changes

### *Exam*

- Motor and sensory deficits

### *Testing*

- MRI is used for early diagnosis and prognosis.
- CT
- CSF demonstrates increased protein.

### *Pitfalls*

- Misdiagnosis
- Typically there is no change with discectomy.

## Red Flags

- None acutely

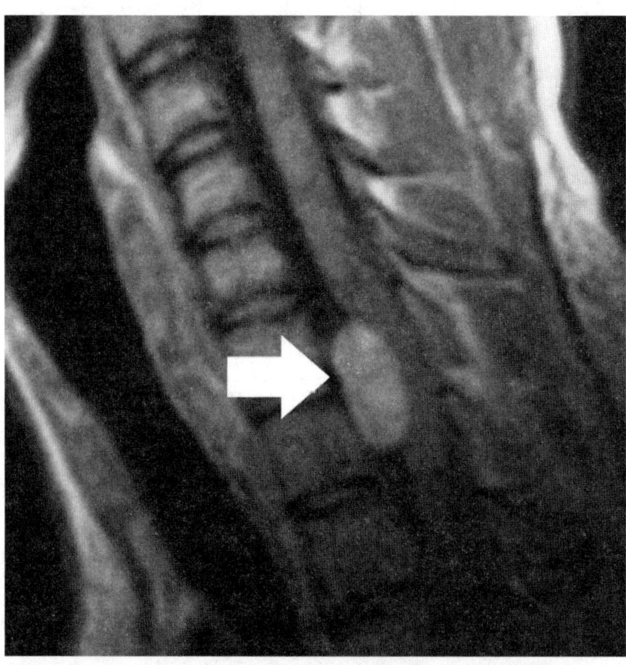

Sagittal T1-weighted magnetic resonance image with contrast demonstrating a schwannoma at the C7–T1 level (arrow). (Adapted from Fast A, Goldsher D. *Navigating the Adult Spine: Bridging Clinical Practice and Neuroradiology*. New York: Demos Medical Publishing, 2007:115.)

## Treatment

### Medical

- None

### Exercises

- None

### Modalities

- None

### Injection

- None

### Surgical

- Resection possible
- Radiation therapy

### Consults

- Neurologic or orthopedic-spine surgery
- Radiation oncology

### Complications of treatment

- Continued neurologic dysfunction following surgical resection
- Spinal instability related to surgical resection
- Arachnoiditis with surgery

## Prognosis

- Usually excellent recovery following a complete resection, although there is a risk of recurrence.

## Helpful Hints

- Possible misdiagnosis

## Suggested Readings

Conti P, Pansini G, Mouchaty H, Capuano C, Conti R. Spinal neurinomas: retrospective analysis and long-term outcome of 179 consecutively operated cases and review of the literature. *Surg Neurol.* 2004;61(1):34–43.

Guyer RD, Collier RR, Ohnmeiss DD, et al. Extraosseous spinal lesions mimicking disc disease. *Spine.* 1988;13(3):328–331.

Nicoletti GF, Passanisi M, Castana L, Albanese V. Intramedullary spinal neurinoma: case report and review of 46 cases. *J Neurosurg Sci.* 1994;38(3):187–191.

# Scoliosis

## Description

Scoliosis is a lateral curvature of the spine greater than 10 degrees.

## Etiology/Types

- Functional scoliosis reduces to normal with forward bending.
- Kyphoscoliosis describes a lateral curvature with an increased sagittal angulation.
- Major categories of adult scoliosis
  - Individuals younger than 40 years without degenerative changes with scoliosis since adolescence
  - Individuals older than 40 years with degenerative changes
  - Elderly individuals who develop scoliosis due to degenerative changes of the thoracolumbar spine
- More than 90% of cases are of an unknown etiology.

## Epidemiology

- Found in up to 7.5% of individuals
- Prevalence increases with age.
- Increased female prevalence with curves >20 degrees

## Pathogenesis

- Generally unknown

## Risk Factors

- Compression fractures related to osteoporosis
- Osteoarthritis
- Possibly genetically related

## Clinical Features

- Pain may be related to zygapophyseal (facet) degeneration, nerve root impingement on the concave side, or rib impingement on the iliac crest.
- Pain worsens with curve progression

## Natural History

- A lumbar curve in a skeletally mature individual <40 degrees will not progress, whereas a curve >40 degrees will progress 1 degree per year.

## Diagnosis

### *Differential diagnosis*

- Congenital diseases
- Extraspinal or hip contractures
- Leg-length discrepancy
- Metabolic disorders
- Nerve root irritation/postural
- Neuromuscular diseases
- Osteomalacia
- Osteoid osteoma
- Rheumatoid disease
- Trauma
- Tumors

### *History*

- Increasing pain just below the apex of the curve
- Pain worsens with activity and improves with recumbency.
- Family history of scoliosis
- Unequal trouser-leg lengths

### *Exam*

- Focus is on shoulder, scapular, and pelvic asymmetry or obliquity as well as leg-length discrepancy.
- Neurologic evaluation to assess for possible nerve root compression
- Pulmonary evaluation should be followed for severely scoliotic patients.

### *Testing*

- Full-length anterior–posterior and lateral thoracolumbar X-rays
- The Cobb method is used to measure the angle of lateral spinal curvature by measuring the angle between two intersecting perpendicular lines that originate from the superior endplate of the upper vertebral body and the inferior endplate of the inferior vertebral body.
- Progression is noted if there is an increase of >5 degrees in the curvature compared to previous films.
- CT and MRI are limited to patients with suspected nerve root involvement or in surgical planning.
- Pulmonary testing

### *Pitfalls*

- Missing a reversible cause of scoliosis such as an osteoid osteoma or a leg-length discrepancy

## Red Flags

- Continued progression of the scoliotic curve
- Pulmonary compromise

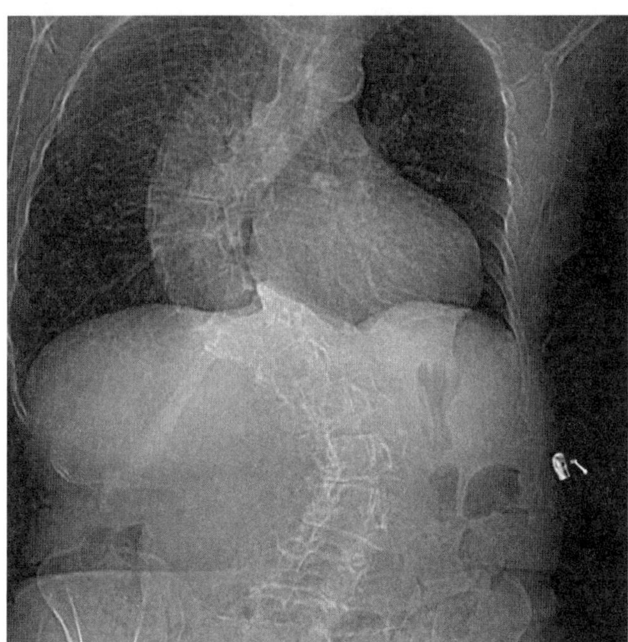

Coronal computed tomography scout film demonstrating severe scoliosis.

## Treatment

### *Medical*

- Heel lift for patients with leg-length discrepancies
- Analgesics
- NSAIDs
- Milwaukee brace for adolescents

### *Exercises*

- General strengthening and stretching exercises
- Yoga has been found to be helpful.

### *Modalities*

- Heat, cold, ultrasound, and transcutaneous electrical nerve stimulation have been used for symptomatic relief of pain and muscle spasms.

### *Injection*

- Zygapophyseal (facet) joint injections for zygapophyseal (facet) joint pain
- Medial branch block testing followed by radiofrequency denervation of the medial branch associated with zygapophyseal (facet) joint pain
- Epidural steroid injection for radicular symptoms

### *Surgical*

- Indicated for progression of scoliosis in patients younger than 40 years if the curve is >50 degrees.
- In those aged 40 years and older, indications include progression, radicular pain, and pulmonary compromise.
- Surgery can restore function in patients.
- Important to assess bone density during preoperative surgical planning

### *Consults*

- Physical medicine and rehabilitation
- Neurologic or orthopedic-spine surgery (clinicians with extensive experience with scoliosis surgery)

### *Complications of treatment*

- Surgical risks include pseudoarthrosis, infection, and the development of curvature above the fusion.

## Prognosis

- Increased morbidity and mortality with untreated severe scoliosis due to increased pain and pulmonary compromise

## Helpful Hints

- A lumbar curve in a skeletally mature individual >40 degrees will progress 1 degree per year.

## Suggested Reading

Lonstein JE. Scoliosis: surgical versus nonsurgical treatment. *Clin Orthop Relat Res.* 2006;443:248–259.

# Spinal Cord Injury

## Description

Spinal cord injury results in the loss of motor and/or sensory function below the level of injury resulting in loss of function of the caudal limbs with bowel and bladder deficits.

## Etiology/Types

- Etiology includes motor vehicle accidents, falls, sports, violence, vascular disorders, infectious causes, vertebral body compression fractures, developmental disorders, and tumors.
- Complete injury describes the loss of motor and sensory function in the lowest sacral segments.
- Incomplete injury describes preservation of sensory and/or motor functions below the level of injury.
- Tetraplegia describes loss of motor and/or sensory function within the cervical spinal cord resulting in impaired function of the arms, trunk, pelvic organs, and legs.
- Paraplegia describes loss of motor and/or sensory function within the spinal cord in the thoracic or lumbar spinal cord or sacral nerve roots resulting in impaired function in the trunk, pelvic organs, and legs.

## Epidemiology

- 12,000 new cases per year in the United States
- Average age of injury is 39.5 years
- Male to female ratio 4:1
- 42% of all injuries result from motor vehicle accidents.
- 23.8% of all injuries result from falls.
- Falls are the most common cause of injury in people over the age of 60.

## Pathogenesis

- Kinetic energy of the injury or trauma causes spinal cord compression with neuronal and vascular injury followed by hemorrhage, inflammation, and ischemia resulting in further damage to the spinal cord.

## Risk Factors

- Caucasian ancestry
- Falls in the elderly population
- Fewer years of education
- Male gender
- Motor vehicle accidents/diving
- Single
- Unemployment
- Violence

## Clinical Features

- Based on presenting level of injury
- Spinal shock lasts an average of 3 weeks and is thought to be due to the interruption of the descending excitatory fibers resulting in the loss of the reflex arc with flaccid muscles.
- Loss of bulbocavernosus reflex during the period of spinal shock
- Increased reflexive activity following spinal shock results from the loss of the descending inhibitory impulses.

## Natural History

- Functional outcome is based on the level of injury.

## Diagnosis

### *Differential diagnosis*

- None for trauma-related spinal cord injury

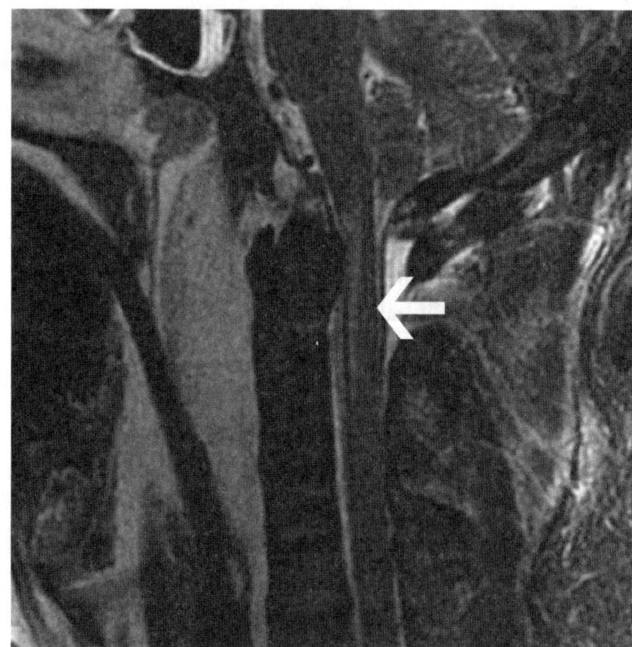

Sagittal cervical T2-weighted magnetic resonance image with fat suppression demonstrating increased signal within the spinal cord at the C0–C2 level (arrow) following a fall from a fifth storey building. (Courtesy of Keith Hentel, MD.)

### History
- Associated injury or trauma with loss of function of the upper or lower extremities with bowel and bladder dysfunction

### Exam
- Based on American Spinal Injury Association (ASIA) classification

### Testing
- Appropriate MRI or CT to assess trauma or injury
- Electrodiagnostic studies to rule out peripheral nerve injury

### Pitfalls
- The physical examination is most accurate 72 hours post-injury, allowing for an initial prognosis.
- Hypercalcemia

## Red Flags
- Missed fractures, peripheral nerve injuries, and traumatic brain injury

## Treatment

### Medical
- Differentiation of neurogenic shock from hypovolemic shock
- Early traction for cervical fractures
- Intravenous methylprednisolone
- Assessment of skin with frequent positioning
- Indwelling urinary catheter

### Exercises
- Range of motion exercises as the patient recovers from spinal shock to prevent contractures

### Modalities
- Heat, cold, ultrasound, and transcutaneous electrical nerve stimulation have been used for symptomatic relief of pain and muscle spasms.

### Injection
- None in the acute setting

### Surgical
- Optimal timing for surgery is believed to be within 24 hours of injury.

### Consults
- Physical medicine and rehabilitation
- Neurologic or orthopedic-spine surgery

### Complications during acute rehabilitation
- Autonomic dysreflexia
- Orthostatic hypotension
- Bowel and bladder dysfunction
- 16% to 53% of patients develop heterotropic ossification.
- 47% to 100% of patients develop a deep vein thrombosis.
- 11% to 94% of patients develop pain.
- Gastric atony and ileus in the acute phase
- Pneumonia/pulmonary embolism
- Spasticity
- Pressure ulcers

## Prognosis
- Prognosis is most accurate after 72 hours, after which a complete injury rarely becomes an incomplete injury.
- Preservation of pinprick sensation below the level of injury at 72 hours postinjury increases the chances of progression to ASIA status D or E.
- Patients with complete tetraplegia may regain at least one motor level within the first 1 to 2 years.
- Patients with three-fifths of quadriceps strength at 2 months postinjury may walk by 1 year postinjury.

## Helpful Hints
- The physical examination is most predictive within 72 hours of injury.

## Suggested Reading
Branco F, Cardenas DD, Svircev JN. Spinal cord injury: a comprehensive review. *Phys Med Rehabil Clin N Am.* 2007;18(4):651–679.

# Spinal Stenosis, Cervical (Cervical Myelopathy)

## Description

Cervical spinal stenosis is the most common spinal cord dysfunction in the older population and is the most common cause of nontraumatic spastic paraparesis and tetraparesis.

## Etiology/Types

- Extensive degenerative changes in the axial spine can cause spinal cord ischemia at one or more levels.

## Epidemiology

- Unknown

## Pathogenesis

- Spondylotic changes result from disc degeneration increasing mechanical stress at the endplates of adjacent vertebral bodies with the development of osteophytic spurs.
- Osteophytic spurs increase the weight-bearing surface of the endplates stabilizing the adjacent vertebrae and decreasing the hypermobility, which results from disc degeneration.
- With cervical flexion, the spinal cord lengthens and is stretched over the ventral osteophytic bars.

## Risk Factors

- Congenital central stenosis
- Down syndrome
- Repeated occupational trauma

## Clinical Features

- Gait abnormality
- Lower-extremity weakness and spasticity
- No pain associated with progression
- Loss of manual dexterity
- Triceps and/or hand intrinsic weakness is common in the upper extremity.
- Iliopsoas and quadriceps muscle weakness is common in the lower extremities.
- Changes in bowel or bladder function may occur at later stages.

## Natural History

- Slow and insidious progression of symptoms

## Diagnosis

### *Differential diagnosis*

- Amyotrophic lateral sclerosis
- Multiple sclerosis
- Polyneuropathy
- Primary lateral sclerosis
- Radiculopathy
- Rheumatoid arthritis
- Spinal arteriovenous malformations
- Spinal cord tumor
- Syringomyelia
- Tabes dorsalis

### *History*

- Upper- or lower-extremity weakness, numbness, or tingling
- Difficulty with fine motor control
- Gait abnormality due to lower extremity weakness and/or proprioceptive deficits

### *Exam*

- Lhermitte's sign resulting in electrical shocks down the trunk and extremities with flexion of the cervical spine
- Fixed neck flexion
- Weakness in affected dermatomes

### *Testing*

- X-rays can be difficult to interpret as cervical spondylotic changes increase with aging.
- An anterior–posterior canal diameter of <14 mm is abnormal.
- Torg ratio of <0.80 to 0.70 indicates significant cervical spinal stenosis.
- MRI is the best imaging technique for initial screening as it allows for excellent resolution of the spinal cord and subarachnoid space in the cervical spine.
- CT allows better visualization of the bony anatomy and the neural foramen and can be more sensitive for osteophytes and degenerative bony changes.
- Electrodiagnostic studies can be used to rule out a peripheral neuropathy.
- Serial SSEPs may be used for prognosis.

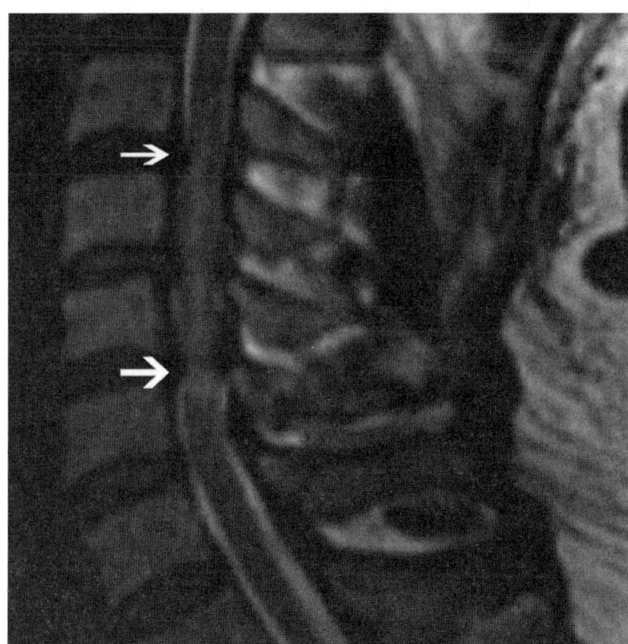

Sagittal cervical T2-weighted magnetic resonance image demonstrating a narrowed central canal and increased signal from C3 to C6 (arrows) resulting in cervical spondylotic myelopathy. (Adapted from Fast A, Goldsher D. *Navigating the Adult Spine: Bridging Clinical Practice and Neuroradiology.* New York: Demos Medical Publishing, 2007:47.)

### *Pitfalls*

- The initial deterioration may be followed by a stable period, in which functional deficits do not progress for many years.

## Red Flags

- Older patients deteriorate more rapidly.

## Treatment

### *Medical*

- Education should include possible complications of disease progression and lifestyle changes to decrease cervical extension.

### *Exercises*

- Rehabilitation is focused on gait and fear of falls as well as activities of daily living, including lifting.

### *Modalities*

- Heat, cold, ultrasound, and transcutaneous electrical nerve stimulation have been used for symptomatic relief of pain and muscle spasms.

### *Injection*

- Epidural steroid injections for radicular symptoms

### *Surgical*

- Surgery is reserved for patients who demonstrate significant functional decline and may allow for functional improvement.

### *Consults*

- Neurologic or orthopedic-spine surgery
- Physical medicine and rehabilitation

### *Complications of treatment*

- Aggressive physical therapy may speed up the functional decline.

## Prognosis

- Disease progression may result in paralysis, bowel or bladder dysfunction, and/or chronic pain.

## Helpful Hints

- Compression in the upper cervical spine (C2–C4) can be suggested by the pectoralis muscle reflex, which is elicited by tapping on the seventh rib between the anterior and middle axillary lines with the arm in abduction.

## Suggested Reading

Baron EM, Young WF. Cervical spondylotic myelopathy: A brief review of its pathophysiology, clinical course, and diagnosis. *Neurosurgery.* 2007;60(suppl 1): S35–S41.

# Spinal Stenosis, Lumbar

## Description

Lumbar spinal stenosis is a narrowing of the central spinal canal. It is a relatively rare condition that presents with single or multiple radiculopathies or myelopathic-like symptoms.

## Etiology/Types

- Degenerative
- Congenital
- Postsurgical

## Epidemiology

- Prevalence increases with age

## Pathogenesis

- Congenital abnormalities include shortened pedicles.
- Degenerative changes first affect the intervertebral disc followed by the zygapophyseal (facet) joints resulting in a thickened ligamentum flavum causing encroachment into the central spinal canal.
- Symptoms are thought to be related to mechanical compression of the neural fibers or reduced blood flow causing hypoxia and perineural fibrosis.

## Risk Factors

- Congenitally small spinal canal
- Genetic predisposition

## Clinical Features

- Clinical diagnosis
- Pseudoclaudication describes buttock, thigh, and leg pain that worsens with walking or standing and improves with sitting.
- "Shopping cart" sign describes improvement in symptoms observed when patient pushes a shopping cart in forward flexion.

## Natural History

- The natural course of lumbar stenosis is one of stable symptoms or improvement with no deterioration based on a 4-year prospective trial.

## Diagnosis

### *Differential diagnosis*

- Achondroplasia
- Amyloid deposition
- Calcium pyrophosphate crystal deposition
- Intraspinal tumors
- Lateral recess stenosis
- Osteoporosis with fracture
- Paget's disease
- Radiculopathy
- Scoliosis
- Trauma

### *History*

- Deep dull ache in the buttocks and posterior legs
- Pain with walking or standing and relief with sitting or bending forward
- Pain may also be improved with leaning over or walking uphill.

### *Exam*

- Motor weakness, atrophy, and asymmetric deep tendon reflexes
- Some clinicians have patients walk until symptoms occur.
- Wide-based gait
- Thigh pain after 30 seconds of lumbar extension
- Often physical exam findings are difficult to differentiate from age-expected changes.

### *Testing*

- Electrodiagnostic studies may reveal radiculopathy or bilateral multisegmental denervation and is useful in ruling out peripheral neuropathies and peripheral nerve entrapments.
- X-rays usually demonstrate nonspecific spondylosis, intervertebral disc space narrowing, or degenerative spondylolisthesis, which is most common at the L4–L5 level.
- CT is useful in demonstrating bony canal encroachment from zygapophyseal (facet) joints, disc prolapse, and calcification of the ligamentum flavum as well as the lateral recesses and nerve root canals.
- MRI is the preferred study to assess lumbar spinal stenosis as it can demonstrate the bony and soft tissue structures that may be contributing to the stenotic pattern.
- Treadmill test

### *Pitfalls*

- Missed unassociated radiculopathy

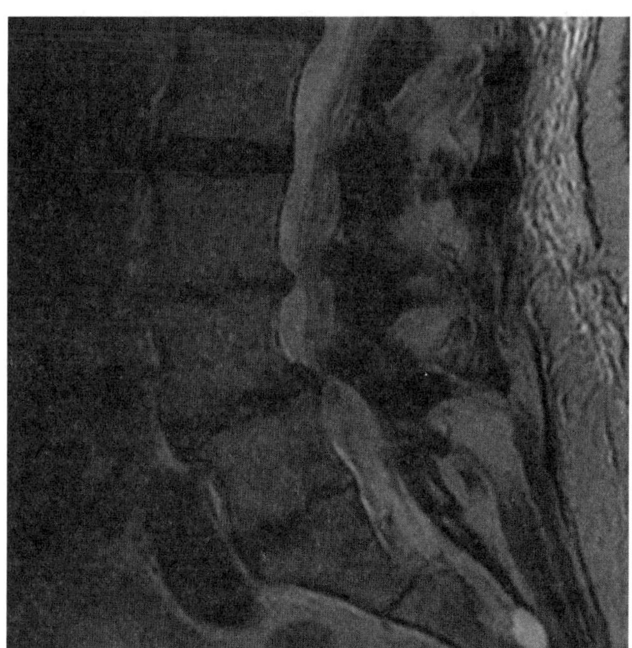

Sagittal lumbar T2-weighted magnetic resonance image demonstrating central spinal stenosis at the L4–L5 level due to anterolisthesis and ligamentum flavum hypertrophy.

## Red Flags

- Bowel or bladder dysfunction
- Gait dysfunction

## Treatment

### *Medical*

- The majority may be treated nonsurgically
- NSAIDs
- Oral prednisone taper

### *Exercises*

- Functional rehabilitation with activity modification, postural training, flexion exercises, conditioning using a stationary exercise bike, and use of aquatic programs

### *Modalities*

- Heat, cold, ultrasound, and transcutaneous electrical nerve stimulation have been used for symptomatic relief of pain and muscle spasms.

### *Injection*

- Up to three fluoroscopically guided epidural steroid injections within a 6-month period can be very effective in relieving symptoms.

### *Surgical*

- Best outcomes with leg pain compared with back pain
- Up to 67% of patients have good to excellent results with a single decompressive surgery.
- 73% of patients followed for 10 years after a laminectomy developed recurrent spinal stenosis.

### *Consults*

- Physical medicine and rehabilitation
- Neurosurgery or orthopedic-spine surgery

### *Complications of treatment*

- Complications related to epidural steroid injections
- Complications related to surgery

## Prognosis

- Initial conservative therapy is appropriate and does not reduce the chance of a good future surgical outcome.

## Helpful Hints

- The diagnosis of spinal stenosis should rely less on absolute radiographic values and more on the relative space and configuration at each level.

## Suggested Reading

Rittenberg JD, Ross AE. Functional rehabilitation for degenerative lumbar spinal stenosis. *Phys Med Rehabil Clin N Am.* 2003;14(1):111–120.

# Spinal Stenosis, Thoracic (Thoracic Myelopathy)

## Description

Thoracic spinal stenosis is the narrowing of the central spinal canal, a relatively rare condition that presents with radiculopathy or myelopathy.

## Etiology/Types

- Caused by degenerative spine disease

## Epidemiology

- Unknown

## Pathogenesis

- Congenitally narrowed thoracic canal becomes further narrowed by a disc herniation, hypertrophy of the posterior elements, ossification or hypertrophy of the ligamentum flavum, ossification or hypertrophy of the posterior longitudinal ligament, and ventral epidural osteophytes.
- Ligamentum flavum ossification tends to affect the lower thoracic spine.
- Posterior longitudinal ligament and ligamentum flavum ossification tend to affect the upper and middle thoracic spine.
- The thoracic spinal canal contains the lumbosacral cord enlargement as well as the lower thoracic to sacral nerve roots, resulting in mixed upper and lower motor neuron presentations.
- 2% of patients with thoracic disc herniations have associated central canal stenosis.

## Risk Factors

- Developmental and acquired narrowing of the thoracic spinal canal
- Mild or moderate traumatic injury

## Clinical Features

- Congenital narrowing predisposes patients to a more abrupt onset of symptoms.
- Unilateral or bilateral pseudoclaudication
- Focal radicular pain or paresthesias
- Symptoms develop due to physical exercise or prolonged kyphotic posturing.

## Natural History

- With progression, bowel and bladder dysfunction and gait abnormality.

## Diagnosis

### *Differential diagnosis*

- Achondroplasia
- Acromegaly
- Ankylosing spondylitis
- Charcot disease related to diabetes or syphilis
- Concurrent symptomatic cervical and lumbar spinal canal stenosis
- Chondro-osteodystrophy
- Diffuse idiopathic skeletal hyperostosis
- Familial hypophosphatemic vitamin D; refractory rickets
- Hemangiomas
- Infection
- Multiple sclerosis
- Osteofluorosis
- Paget's disease
- Renal osteodystrophy
- Scheuermann's disease
- Spinal tumors or cysts
- Spinal vascular malformations

### *History*

- Progressive weakness and numbness
- Decreased balance
- Decreased ability to walk
- Bowel or bladder dysfunction
- Lower-extremity fatigue, tightness, cramping
- Symptoms may develop in one leg then progress to the other.

### *Exam*

- May be normal
- Posterior column dysfunction and upper motor neuron signs may appear with progression.

### *Testing*

- MRI
- CT or CT-myelogram
- Electrodiagnostic studies

### Pitfalls

- Neglecting to consider thoracic spinal stenosis in patients with no evidence of cervical and/or lumbar spinal stenosis

## Red Flags

- Progressive myelopathy
- Progressive bowel or bladder dysfunction

## Treatment

### Medical

- None

### Exercises

- General strengthening and stretching
- Aerobic conditioning
- Gait and balance training

### Modalities

- Heat, cold, ultrasound, and transcutaneous electrical nerve stimulation have been used for symptomatic relief of pain and muscle spasms.

### Injection

- Fluoroscopically guided intralaminar thoracic epidural steroid injection

### Surgical

- Surgical indication includes significant progressive myelopathy with neuroimaging correlation.
- An anterior approach, transpedicular, transfacetal, or costotransversectomy for a disc herniation or ventral osteophyte
- Thoracic laminectomy for posterior disease affecting the zygapophyseal (facet) joints or ligamentum flavum

### Consults

- Physical medicine and rehabilitation
- Neurologic or orthopedic-spine surgery

### Complications of treatment

- Complications related to epidural steroid injections
- Surgical complications include wound infection, cerebrospinal fluid leak, epidural hematoma, iatrogenic spinal instability

## Prognosis

- Untreated myelopathy may progress to bowel and bladder dysfunction and gait abnormalities.
- Surgical treatment may be able to resolve symptoms in the short term.
- Long-term follow-up on surgical patients demonstrates less optimal results due to recurrent stenosis or instability.

## Helpful Hints

- Follow changes in symptomatology focused on acute changes

## Suggested Readings

Botwin KP, Baskin M, Rao S. Adverse effects of fluoroscopically guided interlaminar thoracic epidural steroid injections. *Am J Phys Med Rehabil.* 2006;85(1):14–23.

Rosenbloom SA. Thoracic disc disease and stenosis. *Radiol Clin North Am.* 1991;29(4):765–775.

# Spondylolysis/Spondylolisthesis, Cervical

## Description

Cervical spondylolysis is a bony defect between the superior and inferior articular zygapophyseal (facet) joints of the articular pillar.

Spondylolisthesis refers to a slippage of the vertebra relative to the adjacent vertebra and can result from spondylolysis.

## Etiology/Types

- Spondylolysis is thought to be of a congenital origin or repetitive microtrauma.
- Spondylolisthesis is thought to be related to spondylolysis or age-related changes.

## Epidemiology

- Spondylolysis with or without spondylolisthesis is rare.
- 70% of reported cases involve the C6 vertebra as it is a transitional vertebra between the cervical and thoracic sections.
- Reported at every level except C1 and C7
- Male to female ratio of 2:1
- Age ranges from 5 to 60 years
- Left side more predominant in unilateral cases
- Bilateral involvement occurs in two-thirds of cases.

## Pathogenesis

- The congenital origin of spondylolysis is based on incomplete fusion of the cartilaginous ring due to failure to unite the lateral and posterior ring chondrification centers.
- Spondylolisthesis is thought to be related to the degenerative cascade resulting in zygapophyseal (facet) joint arthrosis and disc degeneration.
- Trauma

## Risk Factors

- Spondylolisthesis—advanced age, aneurysmal bone cyst, neurofibromatosis
- Spondylolysis—spina bifida, laminae dysplasia

## Clinical Features

- Often asymptomatic
- Generally first noted during routine trauma imaging
- Frequently associated with radiculopathy
- Spinal cord compression is uncommon.
- 59% of patients have a grade 1 spondylolisthesis.
- 59% have associated spina bifida.

## Natural History

- Unknown

## Diagnosis

### *Differential diagnosis*

- Dislocation
- Fracture

### *History*

- Neck pain
- Neck rigidity
- Often associated with radicular symptoms

### *Exam*

- Decreased neck range of motion
- Possible neurologic dysfunction may be noted

### *Testing*

- Lateral and oblique X-rays and CT demonstrate a well delineated cleft between the zygapophyseal (facet) joints, a triangular-shaped pillar fragment on either side, posterior displacement of the dorsal fragment, hypoplasia of the ipsilateral pedicle.

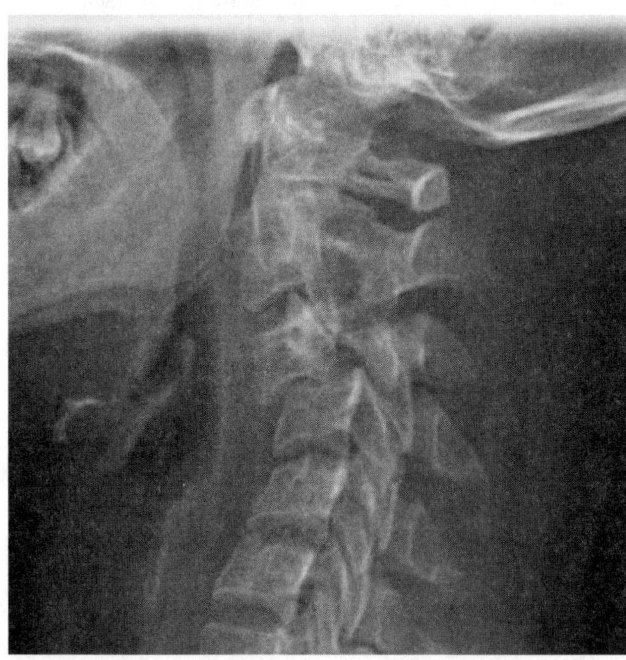

Lateral cervical plain radiograph demonstrating an anterolisthesis of C3 on C4 following a motor vehicle accident. (Courtesy of Keith Hentel, MD.)

- MRI is not helpful unless there is interest in the soft tissues.
- Flexion/extension lateral X-rays are used to assess for instability related to spondylolisthesis.

### *Pitfalls*

- Differentiating a congenital spondylolytic abnormality from an acute fracture or dislocation, which requires emergent surgery during a routine trauma workup

## Red Flags

- Symptoms or signs of spinal cord compression or radiographic instability

## Treatment

### *Medical*

- Often treated conservatively with yearly imaging to assess for possible progression
- NSAIDs
- Soft collar

### *Exercises*

- General neck range of motion and strengthening

### *Modalities*

- Heat, cold, ultrasound, and transcutaneous electrical nerve stimulation have been used for symptomatic relief of pain and muscle spasms.

### *Injection*

- None

### *Surgical*

- Reserved for those who fail conservative management or develop neurologic compromise due to instability
- Anterior or posterior interbody fusion

### *Consults*

- Physical medicine and rehabilitation
- Neurologic or orthopedic-spine surgery

### *Complications of treatment*

- Complications related to epidural steroid injections
- Complications related to surgery

## Prognosis

- Conservative treatment can result in complete resolution of spondylolytic symptoms.
- A wrestler was able to return to national competition within 2 years of surgery for a spondylolytic defect.

## Helpful Hints

- Remember the challenge of differentiating a congenital abnormality from an acute fracture or dislocation

## Suggested Readings

Oueslati S, Zaouia K, Chelli M. Cervical spondylolysis: a case report. *Acta Orthop Belg.* 2006;72(4):511–516.

Pitzen T, Johann K, Steudel WI, Fritsch E. Cervical spondylolisthesis C6–C7 in a young wrestler: case report. *Zentralbl Neurochir.* 2008;69(2):96–98.

Woiciechowsky C, Thomale UW, Kroppenstedt SN. Degenerative spondylolisthesis of the cervical spine—symptoms and surgical strategies depending on disease progress. *Eur Spine J.* 2004;13(8):680–684.

# Spondylolysis/Spondylolisthesis, Lumbar

## Description

Spondylolysis refers to a defect in the pars interarticularis. Spondylolisthesis refers to a slippage of the vertebra relative to the adjacent vertebra.

## Etiology/Types

- Spondylolysis often leads to a spondylolisthesis.
- Congenital spondylolisthesis
  - Dysplastic allows for the anterior translation of a vertebra on the adjacent vertebra
  - Isthmic involves a pars interarticularis lesion, most commonly at the L5 level
- Acquired spondylolisthesis
  - Degenerative
  - Traumatic
  - Pathologic related to a tumor
- Meyerding spondylolisthesis grading system
  - Grade 1 is up to 25% of translation.
  - Grade 2 is 26% to 50%.
  - Grade 3 is 51% to 75%.
  - Grade 4 is 76% to 100%
  - Grade 5 is >100% also known as spondyloptosis.

## Epidemiology

- Spondylolysis occurs in 15% to 70% of first-degree relatives.
- Spondylolysis is reported to have a male to female ratio of 2:1.
- In general, spondylolisthesis is reported to have a male to female ratio of 1:2–3.

## Pathogenesis

- Repetitive or traumatic lumbar extension results in a stress fracture of the pars interarticularis.
- Degenerative spondylolisthesis is most common at the L4–L5 level followed by the L3–L4 level.

## Risk Factors

- American football and gymnastics
- Pregnancy
- The risk of slip progression is increases with higher grades of spondylolisthesis and higher slip angles.

## Clinical Features

- Lumbar hyperlordosis
- High-grade spondylolysis may be noted with a palpable step-off deformity or a dimple
- Increased pain with lumbar hyperextension
- Hamstring tightness thought to be associated, with an attempt to stabilize the L5–S1 junction

## Natural History

- 15% of individuals have progression of their spondylolysis to spondylolisthesis with no evidence of worsening back pain.
- The slippage is usually noted during the growth spurt with decreased progression every 10 years.

## Diagnosis

### *Differential diagnosis*

- Lower back sprain or strain
- Peripheral neuropathy
- Vascular insufficiency

### *History*

- Low back pain
- Lower-extremity pain
- Assess for an associated radiculopathy in high-grade slippage (>50%)
- Pain worsens with activity and improves with rest

### *Exam*

- Positive stork test or single-leg standing hyperextension test
- Flattened lumbar lordosis with muscle spasm
- Pelvic waddle gait described as a stiff-legged gait with short strides
- Dural root tension signs
- Palpable step-off deformity

### *Testing*

- Oblique X-rays demonstrate a broken neck or collar of the "Scotty dog" confirming a pars interarticularis fracture.
- Flexion extension X-rays are useful to asses for anterior–posterior instability.
- Lateral X-rays are useful to assess the degree of translation, the sacral inclination, slip angle.
- Instability is considered with slips on lateral X-rays of >50%.
- SPECT can localize the level of the lesion, and increased activity suggests healing potential.
- Thin-cut tomography may demonstrate the fracture and is useful for follow-up evaluations.

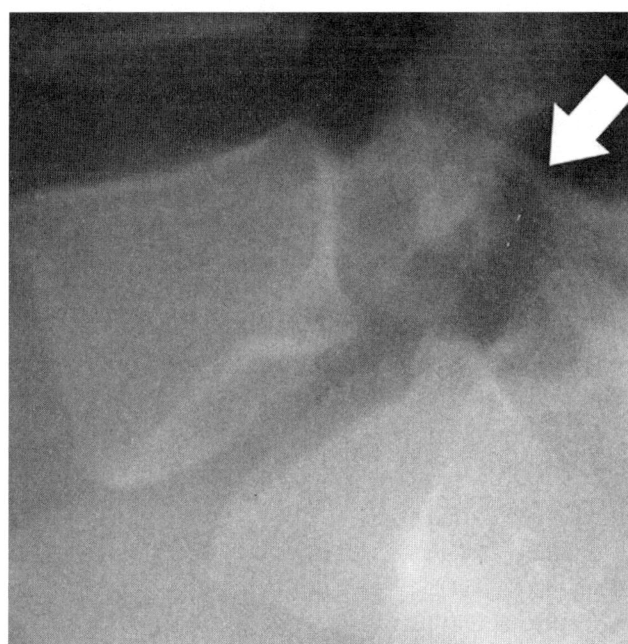

Lateral lumbar plain radiograph demonstrating a grade 1 anterolisthesis and a defect in the pars interarticularis (arrow) at the L5–S1 level. (Adapted from Fast A, Goldsher D. *Navigating the Adult Spine: Bridging Clinical Practice and Neuroradiology*. New York: Demos Medical Publishing, 2007:56.)

- MRI to evaluate for a stress response and potential radiculopathy

### *Pitfalls*

- Diagnostic difficulty for spondylolysis

## Red Flags

- Neurologic compromise

## Treatment

### *Medical*

- Cessation of sporting activities
- NSAIDs
- Spinal orthosis

### *Exercises*

- Hip flexion and hamstring contracture stretching
- Core lumbar stabilization

### *Modalities*

- Heat, cold, ultrasound, and transcutaneous electrical nerve stimulation have been used for symptomatic relief of pain and muscle spasms.

### *Injection*

- Blocks of the pars interarticularis may be helpful in diagnosis and treatment.

### *Surgical*

- L5–S1 fusion with autologous posterior iliac crest bone graft for symptomatic L5 spondylolysis
- Decompression is considered in patients with radiculopathy or bowel or bladder dysfunction.

### *Consults*

- Physical medicine and rehabilitation
- Neurologic or orthopedic-spine surgery

### *Complications of treatment*

- Complications related to injection and surgery

## Prognosis

- Patients may heal spontaneously
- Patients with symptoms should refrain from heavy lifting or high-level athletic activities.
- No heavy lifting or high-level athletic activities following surgical fusion

## Helpful Hints

- Assessment for neurologic compromise

## Suggested Reading

Hu SS, Tribus CB, Diab M, Ghanayem AJ. Spondylolisthesis and spondylolysis. *J Bone Joint Surg Am*. 2008;90(3):656–671.

# Spontaneous Epidural Hematoma

## Description

Acute bleeding into the epidural space of the spinal canal

## Etiology/Types

- Most occur spontaneously
- Acute bleeding from an extradural vessel or the posterior epidural venous plexus
- Chronic types are rare and typically occur in the cervical spine.

## Epidemiology

- Spontaneous hematomas account for up to 50% of all spinal epidural hematomas.
- Most common in patients 50 to 80 years of age
- Most common in the cervicothoracic spine, followed by the thoracolumbar spine
- Cervical spine more commonly involved in children and young adults
- Male to female ratio is 1.5:1

## Pathogenesis

- The lumbar spine is better able to accommodate to an expanding mass due to its larger diameter.
- Extends for at least two or more segments
- Found most commonly in the posterolateral position
- Sudden nerve root or spinal cord compression
- Sudden compression of the anterior spinal artery

## Risk Factors

- Anticoagulation
- Arteriovenous malformations
- Chiropractic spinal manipulation
- Cocaine use
- Hemophilia
- Leukemia
- Myelography
- Spinal procedures
- Spondylosis
- Surgery
- Thrombocytopenia

## Clinical Features

- Sudden and severe neck or back pain
- Radicular pain
- Neurologic dysfunction
- Bowel or bladder dysfunction
- Symptoms may progress from minutes to hours.
- Other presentations include slowly progressive, chronic, and relapsing symptoms.

## Natural History

- Sudden and progressive radiculopathy or spinal cord injury

## Diagnosis

### *Differential diagnosis*

- Epidural abscess
- Intervertebral disc herniation
- Lumbar spinal stenosis

### *History*

- Initial symptoms may be vague
- Sudden and severe neck or back pain
- Motor and sensory dysfunction
- Bowel or bladder dysfunction

### *Exam*

- Motor and sensory dysfunction
- Bowel or bladder dysfunction

### *Testing*

- MRI demonstrates a mass that is isodense on T1-weighted images with increased signal on T2-weighted images within the first 24 hours. After 24 hours, there is high T1-weighted signal and low T2-weighted signal.
- MRI with contrast may demonstrate peripheral enhancement or occasional central enhancement.

### *Pitfalls*

- Delayed treatment

## Red Flags

- Progressive motor and sensory dysfunction
- Bowel or bladder dysfunction

## Treatment

### *Medical*

- Indicated with mild presentations, serious coagulopathy, high operative risks, or prolonged paralysis
- Anticoagulated patients may receive vitamin K and fresh frozen plasma.

- Platelet transfusion with thrombocytopenia
- Treatment of coagulopathy may prevent progression of the hematoma and allow for nonoperative treatment as some believe that the hematoma remains as liquid longer in patients with coagulopathies, allowing it to spread further along the epidural space.
- Cervical epidural hematoma may respond to neck immobilization and steroid administration.

### *Exercises*

- None

### *Modalities*

- None

### *Injection*

- None

### *Surgical*

- Emergent decompressive laminectomy with hematoma evacuation is considered with neurologic dysfunction.

### *Consults*

- Neurologic and orthopedic-spine surgery

### *Complications of treatment*

- Radiculopathy
- Spinal cord injury
- Death

## Prognosis

- Best outcomes are observed if the surgery is completed within 36 hours with complete SCI injuries and ≤48 hours with incomplete SCI injuries.
- Based on extent of the hematoma, the preoperative neurologic deficits, and the time interval between symptom onset and surgical decompression
- Lumbar hematomas have the best prognosis.
- Cervical and thoracic hematomas have a poorer outcome.
- Incomplete sensory and motor deficits suggest a good postoperative recovery.
- Preoperative absence of sensorimotor function does not indicate a poor outcome.
- Cervical or cervicothoracic presentations may favor spontaneous recovery.

## Helpful Hints

- Always include a spontaneous epidural hematoma in the differential of acute neck or low back pain.

## Suggested Readings

Liu WH, Hsieh CT, Chiang YH, Chen GJ. Spontaneous spinal epidural hematoma of thoracic spine: a rare case report and review of literature. *Am J Emerg Med.* 2008;26(3):384.e1–2.

Groen RJ. Non-operative treatment of spontaneous spinal epidural hematomas: a review of the literature and a comparison with operative cases. *Acta Neurochir* (Wien). 2004;146(2):103–110.

# Stingers and Burners

## Description

Stingers and burners describe cervical nerve root or brachial plexus injuries resulting in shoulder and upper-extremity pain, dysesthesias, and weakness.

## Etiology/Types

- Traction: lateral neck flexion to the contralateral side with ipsilateral shoulder depression
- Compression: shoulder pad compression of the brachial plexus against the superior medial scapula at Erb's point
- Hyperextension with or without lateral flexion: nerve root compression within the intervertebral foramen
- Shoulder distraction away from the neck or forced oblique neck extension

## Epidemiology

- Thought to be the most common injury in sports medicine, although commonly under-reported
- 18% to 65% of collegiate football players experience this condition.

## Pathogenesis

- C5 and C6 anterior rami make up the upper trunk and converge at Erb's point making it the most commonly injured region.
- Cervical nerve roots are susceptible to injury due to
  - lack of a protective epineurium, perineurium
  - dural dentate ligaments that anchor roots
  - compression of the nerve roots between the vertebral artery and the transverse process or due to scalene muscle hypertrophy.
- C4–C5 and C5–C6 foramen are most commonly affected.

## Risk Factors

- Basketball, boxing, weightlifting, rugby
- Degenerative changes of the cervical spine
- Football is the most common cause.
- Wrestling is the second most common cause.

## Clinical Features

- Stinging or burning-type pain radiating with possible weakness affecting the shoulder down the upper limb to the hand
- Athletes shake affected hand
- Associated weakness, numbness, or tingling is found in the affected dermatome
- Neck pain is uncommon.

## Natural History

- Usually self-limiting, lasting from seconds to weeks
- Some cases may lead to persistent subtle neurologic deficits or complete loss of affected extremity function.

## Diagnosis

### *Differential diagnosis*

- Cervical fracture
- Cervical sprain or strain
- Clavicle fracture
- Zygapophyseal (facet) joint dislocation
- Intervertebral disc injury
- Spinal cord injury
- Thoracic outlet syndrome with medial or lower cord changes of the brachial plexus

### *History*

- Burning pain and dysesthesias along a dermatomal pattern
- Shoulder abduction relief sign

### *Exam*

- Rule out possible head injury or spinal cord injury
- Removal of sporting equipment if appropriate
- Assess for swelling, tenderness or deformity
- Active neck range of motion
- Gentle Spurling's maneuver
- Motor, sensory, and reflex testing
- Assess acromioclavicular joint, glenohumeral joint, and supraclavicular region deformity
- Tinel's sign at Erb's point
- Slightly flexed cervical spine posture to decrease pressure within the neuroforamen

### *Testing*

- X-rays of the cervical spine
- Three times greater risk of a burner with a Torg/Pavlov ratio of <0.8, indicating cervical spinal stenosis
- MRI can be used to assess brachial plexus injury, soft tissue, or spinal cord injury
- Electrodiagnostic studies should be considered if there is no resolution of symptoms within 3 weeks.

### Pitfalls

- Neck pain and bilateral upper extremity symptoms may suggest a cervical spine injury.
- Glenohumeral joint and rotator cuff injury

## Red Flags

- Cervical spine or supraclavicular injuries may result in medial or lower cord brachial plexus injuries.

## Treatment

### Medical

- Mild neurapraxia: Player may return to play if physical examination is normal.
- Moderate neurapraxia: Serial physical examinations up to 2 weeks due to delayed onset of weakness
- Severe neurapraxia with axonotmesis: Further workup; player allowed to return to play if normal physical examination with modification of protective equipment.
- Neurotmesis has no treatment available.

### Exercises

- Restoration of neck range of motion
- Neck and shoulder strengthening
- Postural exercises
- Proprioceptive and sports-specific exercises

### Modalities

- None

### Injection

- Persistent radicular pain may be treated with an epidural steroid injection.

### Surgical

- Considered if no functional return suggesting neurotmesis

### Consults

- Physical medicine and rehabilitation
- Neurologic surgeon specializing in peripheral nerves

### Complications of treatment

- Permanent loss of function in the affected upper extremity
- Tetraparesis or tetraplegia

## Prognosis

- Preganglionic lesions have poor prognosis.
- Postganglionic lesions may be amenable to surgical repair.
- Mild neurapraxia with resolution in seconds to minutes
- Moderate neurapraxia with resolution in minutes to hours
- Severe neurapraxia with axonotmesis may take over 3 weeks for recovery.
- Neurotmesis recovery is unlikely.
- Return to play is contraindicated with continued neurologic deficits, greater than two previous episodes of transient tetraparesis, or findings of cervical myelopathy.

## Helpful Hints

- Traction injuries are less common in athletes with short thick necks.

## Suggested Reading

Feinberg JH. Burners and stingers. *Phys Med Rehabil Clin N Am.* 2000;11(4):771–784.

# Synovial Cysts

## Description

Cysts associated with the zygapophyseal (facet) joints of the spine are often incidental findings, although they can represent spinal segment instability and be symptomatic.

## Etiology/Types

- Zygapophyseal (facet) joint instability results in increased intra-articular pressure causing a herniation of the synovium through a weakened portion of the joint capsule.
- Most common in regions of spinal instability

## Epidemiology

- Most common age group is in the sixth decade
- Age range from 28 to 94 years
- Female to male ratio is 1–4:1
- 88% to 99% occur in the lumbar spine.
- 90% to 100% of patients also have spondylolisthesis or degenerative joint disease of the zygapophyseal (facet) joints.
- 54% of patients demonstrate bilateral cysts, most commonly at the L4–L5 level, which indicates segmental instability.

## Pathogenesis

- The level of occurrence is related to the amount of spinal instability and degenerative spondylosis.
- Usually small cysts that are adjacent or attached to the synovial tissue-lined zygapophyseal (facet) joints.
- Lined with cuboid or pseudostratified columnar epithelium
- Attached to the joint via a narrow isthmus connecting the cystic centers
- Also found in other parts of the body including the knees (Baker's cyst), hips, and elbows

## Risk Factors

- Zygapophyseal (facet) joint degenerative changes, 75% to 90%
- Degenerative spondylolisthesis, 38% to 60%
- Genetic predisposition
- Spinal instability, 60%
- Trauma

## Clinical Features

- Often asymptomatic
- Most commonly occurs at the L4–L5 segment, which is the most mobile segment of the lumbar spine, followed in descending order of frequency at the L5–S1, L3–L4, and L2–L3 levels.
- 50% to 93% of cases have low back pain.
- 57% to 100% of cases also have associated radicular symptoms.

## Natural History

- Rarely regresses
- Spontaneous regression reported from 11 weeks to 18 months is thought to be due to cyst rupture.

## Diagnosis

### *Differential diagnosis*

- Arachnoid cyst
- Dermoid cyst
- Ganglion cysts
- Herniated nucleus pulposus
- Meningioma
- Metastatic tumor
- Neurofibroma
- Perineural cyst
- Schwannoma

### *History*

- Low back pain
- Radicular symptoms
- Neurogenic claudication
- Myelopathic symptoms

### *Exam*

- Palpable tenderness over the involved segment
- Radicular or myelopathic signs

### *Testing*

- X-rays can be used to rule out spondylosis, spondylolisthesis, metastatic lesions.
- Cysts are found dorsal, ventromedially to the zygapophyseal (facet) joints, or within the ligamentum flavum.
- MRI demonstrates hypointense masses on T1-weighted images; hyperintense masses on T2-weighted images, which may be hyperintense compared with cerebrospinal fluid.
- CT demonstrates low-density round lesions adjacent to the zygapophyseal (facet) joints, calcifications are occasionally present in the outer walls.

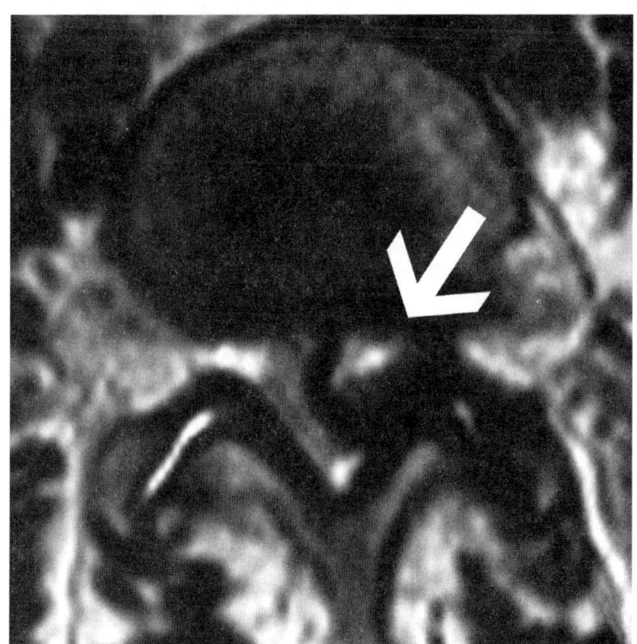

Axial lumbar T2-weighted magnetic resonance image demonstrating a left L5–S1 synovial cyst. (Adapted from Weiner BK, Joel Torretti J, Stauff M. Microdecompression for lumbar synovial cysts: an independent assessment of long term outcomes. *J Orthop Surg Res.* 2007;2:5.)

### *Pitfalls*

- Delayed imaging

## Red Flags

- Unilateral or bilateral radiculopathy
- Neurogenic claudication
- Myelopathy
- Cauda equina syndrome

## Treatment

### *Medical*

- NSAIDs
- Analgesic medications

### *Exercises*

- None

### *Modalities*

- Heat, cold, ultrasound, and transcutaneous electrical nerve stimulation have been used for symptomatic relief of pain and muscle spasms.

### *Injection*

- Epidural steroid injection may relieve the inflammatory component
- Intra-articular zygapophyseal (facet) joint aspiration
- Fluoroscopically or CT-guided translaminar cyst aspiration and puncture

### *Surgical*

- Spinal decompression may include unilateral or bilateral laminotomies, hemilaminectomies or laminectomies, and fusion
- Bilateral cysts indicate segmental instability and a possible need for fusion
- Firmly adherent cysts can make dissection challenging.

### *Consults*

- Physical medicine and rehabilitation
- Neurologic or orthopedic-spine surgery

### *Complications of treatment*

- Complications related to needle aspiration, which include nerve injury
- May recur following needle aspiration or surgery.
- Dural tearing can occur in 4% to 12% of surgical cases.

## Prognosis

- Surgical resection of cysts has resulted in good to excellent results in up to 100% of patients.

## Helpful Hints

- Most symptomatic individuals will eventually require surgery.

## Suggested Reading

Epstein NE. Lumbar synovial cysts: a review of diagnosis, surgical management, and outcome assessment. *J Spinal Disord Tech.* 2004;17(4):321–325.

# Syringomyelia

## Description

Syringomyelia is a fluid-filled cyst lined with glial cells within the central portion of the spinal cord.

## Etiology/Types

- Communicating syringomyelia results from alterations in CSF flow due to obstructive lesions in the foramen magnum.
- Noncommunicating syringomyelia may be idiopathic or associated with traumatic myelopathy, spinal cord tumors, or arachnoiditis.
- Syringomyelia is associated with congenital abnormalities, trauma, infections, or inflammatory abnormalities.

## Epidemiology

- Most common in males ranging in age from 25 to 40 years

## Pathogenesis

- Most common in the cervical spine although occasionally found in the lumbar spine
- Most often extends from below the first cervical segment to the thoracic region spanning seven or more levels
- The cavity is found in the gray matter, posterior to the central canal and contains CSF.

## Risk Factors

- Cervical spinal cord injury
- History of previous lesion removal from the spinal cord

## Clinical Features

- The onset or worsening of symptoms can be brought on by minor trauma.
- Growth results in the loss of pain sensation followed by motor weakness.
- Positive Babinski reflex and other upper motor neuron signs can be found.
- Bowel and bladder dysfunction
- Possible brain stem or cerebellar signs
- Common in patients with cervical spinal cord injuries
- May also occur in patients who have a remote history of surgical removal of lesions from the spinal cord
- 24% of patients report neck pain

## Natural History

- Some patients may not have progression of symptoms whereas others may develop significant functional disability.

## Diagnosis

### *Differential diagnosis*

- Intramedullary neoplasm

### *History*

- Neck pain
- Loss of bilateral pain and temperature sensation

### *Exam*

- Muscle atrophy
- Decreased coordination

### *Testing*

- MRI can localize the syringomyelia and differentiate it from an intramedullary neoplasm.

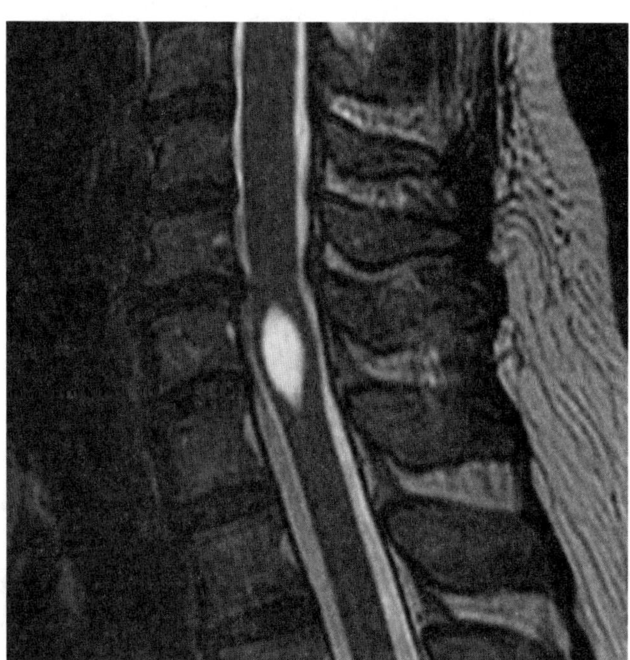

Sagittal cervical T2-weighted magnetic resonance image demonstrating increased signal at the C7–T1 level due to syringomyelia. (Adapted from Fast A, Goldsher D. *Navigating the Adult Spine: Bridging Clinical Practice and Neuroradiology.* New York: Demos Medical Publishing, 2007:137.)

### Pitfalls

- Overlooked progressive functional disability

## Red Flags

- Bowel and bladder dysfunction, spastic paraplegia, infection, arthropathy, progressive functional disability

## Treatment

### Medical

- None

### Exercises

- General strengthening and stretching
- Proprioception and coordination training
- Activities of daily living training

### Modalities

- Heat, cold, ultrasound, and transcutaneous electrical nerve stimulation have been used for symptomatic relief of pain and muscle spasms.

### Injection

- None

### Surgical

- Surgical treatment is based on the progression of symptoms and may include needle aspiration of the fluid, myelotomy, and shunt placement.

### Consults

- Physical medicine and rehabilitation
- Neurologic surgery

### Complications of treatment

- Neuropathic joint disease of the shoulder
- Horner's syndrome
- Complications related to surgery including shunt blockage or infection

## Prognosis

- Up to 22% of patients do not have progression of symptoms over a 20-year period.
- Unchecked progression may result in significant functional disability including spastic paraplegia, infections, or arthropathy.

## Helpful Hints

- Careful monitoring of disease progress is important

## Suggested Readings

Di Lorenzo N, Cacciola F. Adult syringomielia. Classification, pathogenesis and therapeutic approaches. *J Neurosurg Sci.* 2005;49(3):65–72.

Greitz D. Unraveling the riddle of syringomyelia. *Neurosurg Rev.* 2006;29(4):251–263.

# Tarlov Cysts (Perineural Cysts, Sacral Nerve Root Cysts)

## Description

Meningeal dilation of the posterior spinal nerve root sheath that has spinal nerve root fibers within the cyst wall or cavity.

## Etiology/Types

- Cystic formation occurs through infiltrating subarachnoid hemorrhage or trauma-induced intraneural hemorrhage followed by a cystic degeneration of red blood cells and neural tissue destruction.
- Also thought to originate from dural lacerations, increased CSF pressure, congenital dural diverticula, or persistent embryonic fissures.

## Epidemiology

- Found in 4.6% to 9% of the adult population
- Found in the fourth or fifth decade of life
- Female predominant
- Most commonly affects the sacral roots, primarily the S2 and S3 nerve roots
- Only 20% of cysts are symptomatic.

## Pathogenesis

- Located between the perineurium and endoneurium of the posterior nerve root sheath at the dorsal root ganglion

## Risk Factors

- Trauma

## Clinical Features

- May be asymptomatic
- Sacral radiculopathy or pain
- Paresthesias
- Symptoms worsen with standing, coughing, or Valsalva due to subarachnoid pressure, increasing the pressure into the cyst cavity through a "ball and valve" type of communication
- Bowel or bladder dysfunction
- Pain in the perineal region
- Impotence
- Hip, leg, foot pain
- Contralateral symptoms are rare.
- Report of abdominal pain
- Anginalike symptoms from Tarlov cysts in the thoracic spine

## Natural History

- Progressive enlargement resulting in stretching of the sensory nerve roots with compression against the adjacent bone resulting in increased symptoms

## Diagnosis

### *Differential diagnosis*

- Meningeal diverticula

### *History*

- Progressive pain and radiculopathy

### *Exam*

- Positive straight leg raise
- Decreased lumbar flexion

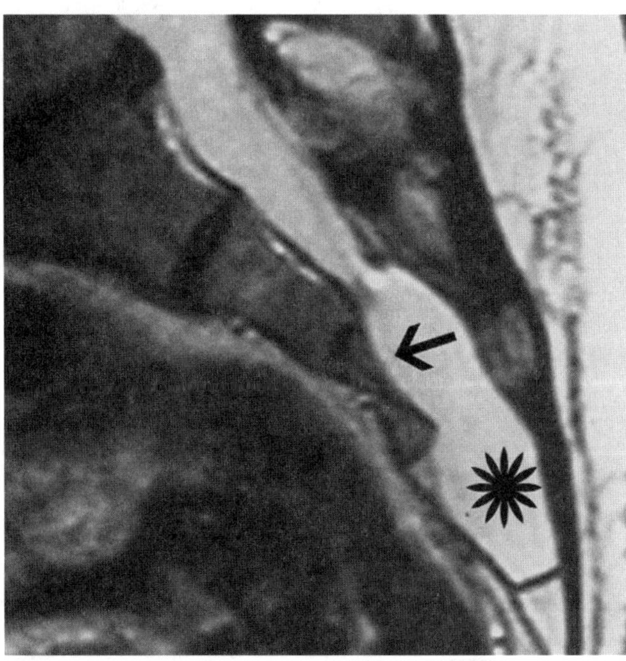

Sagittal lumbosacral T2-weighted magnetic resonance image demonstrating erosion of the sacrum due to a Tarlov cyst (arrow) which is isointense to the cerebrospinal fluid (star). (Adapted from Fast A, Goldsher D. *Navigating the Adult Spine: Bridging Clinical Practice and Neuroradiology*. New York: Demos Medical Publishing, 2007:76.)

### Testing

- X-rays may demonstrate erosion of the sacrum, and rounded paravertebral shadow
- MRI demonstrates CSF-like characteristics, low T1-weighted and high T2-weighted images; may also demonstrate bone and pedicle erosion, neuroformaminal enlargement, or sacral canal widening
- CT demonstrates isodense lesions compared to CSF and bony erosions
- CT myelography may demonstrate a delayed filling pattern of one hour with water-soluble contrast
- Myelography may demonstrate a characteristic delayed filling pattern.
- Electrodiagnostic studies to assess for radiculopathy

### Pitfalls

- Sacral insufficiency fractures may occur due to erosion

## Red Flags

- Bowel or bladder dysfunction
- Impaired mobility

## Treatment

### Medical

- NSAIDs

### Exercises

- Pelvic stabilizers and abdominal muscle strengthening
- Hamstring stretching

### Modalities

- Heat, cold, ultrasound, and transcutaneous electrical nerve stimulation have been used for symptomatic relief of pain and muscle spasms.

### Injection

- Lumbar CSF drainage to decrease CSF pressure and cystic pressure, although symptoms may return once drainage is stopped.
- Percutaneous cyst drainage with use of fibrin glue, although 75% of patients in a study developed aseptic meningitis and procedure may lead to worsening of symptoms due to hemorrhage.
- CT-guided cyst aspiration

### Surgical

- Surgery is recommended if the cyst is >1.5 cm in diameter and patients present with radicular pain.
- Lumboperitoneal shunt for continuous CSF drainage
- Decompressive laminectomy has a low success rate.
- Cyst or nerve root excision leads to significant morbidity.
- Microsurgical cyst fenestration and imbrication with improvement noted up to 17 months

### Consults

- Physical medicine and rehabilitation
- Neurologic or orthopedic-spine surgery

### Complications of treatment

- Potential for recurrence following surgery
- Poor surgical outcomes

## Prognosis

- Variable

## Helpful Hints

- Although most commonly asymptomatic, Tarlov cysts should be considered in a differential diagnosis if other causes have been ruled out.
- Symptoms worsen with standing, coughing, or Valsalva maneuver

## Suggested Reading

Nadler SF, Bartoli LM, Stitik TP, Chen B. Tarlov cyst as a rare cause of S1 radiculopathy: A case report. *Arch Phys Med Rehabil.* 2001;82(5):689–690.

# Tethered Cord Syndrome

## Description

Stretching or tethering of the spinal cord resulting in a traction neuropathy is caused by inelastic structures that may include a fibroadipose filum terminale, myelomeningocele, lipomyelomeningocele, scar tissue, or a bony spicule. First described by Garceau as filum terminale syndrome in 1953.

## Etiology/Types

- Childhood onset is most common.
- Adult delayed onset may be due to cumulative effects of oxidative metabolism impairment, progressive increased filum terminale fibrous tissue with aging, sudden stretching of the spinal cord, or age-related spondylitic changes that exacerbate stretching of the spinal cord.

## Epidemiology

- Unknown

## Pathogenesis

- Oxidative metabolism impairment due to constant stretching of the spinal cord with resulting decreased regional blood flow
- Neuronal membrane changes

## Risk Factors

- Spinal dysraphism

## Clinical Features

- Lower back pain and leg pain that is exacerbated with physical activity, particularly lumbar flexion and extension.
- Groin pain
- Genitorectal pain
- Lower-extremity sensory deficits
- Lower-extremity motor deficits that do not follow a dermatomal pattern
- Muscle atrophy
- Scoliosis
- Increased lumbosacral lordosis
- Sexual dysfunction
- Bladder and bowel dysfunction or incontinence
- Deformities of the lower extremities including pes cavus, pes equines, hammer toes, and leg-length discrepancies
- Gait abnormalities
- Pain
- Cutaneous stigmata include hypertrichosis, a dermal pit, or a subcutaneous lipoma

## Natural History

- Symptoms frequently progress slowly although there may be rapid post-traumatic progression.
- Primarily lower-extremity motor deterioration occurs over years.
- Symptoms exacerbated with prolonged bending or sitting

## Diagnosis

### *Differential diagnosis*

- Disc disease
- Peripheral neuropathy
- Spinal cord tumors
- Spondylolisthesis
- Syringomyelia

### *History*

- Lower-extremity sensorimotor changes
- Bowel or bladder dysfunction

### *Exam*

- Decreased motor function
- Loss of cutaneous sensation
- Spasticity

### *Testing*

- MRI may note a thickened filum terminale (>2 mm diameter), mass, fibroadipose filum terminate, elongated spinal cord, and subarachnoid space obliteration.
- Urodynamics
- Electrodiagnostic studies, including pelvic floor studies
- Somatosensory-evoked potentials

### *Pitfalls*

- Incorrect diagnosis of failed back syndrome or degenerative disc disease
- The symptoms may be gradual, so that patients never seek medical care.

## Red Flags

- Sudden post-traumatic progression

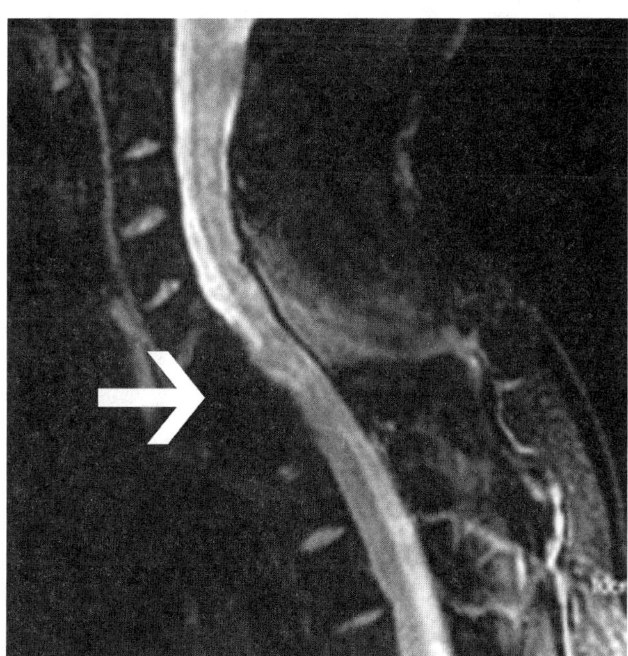

Sagittal cervical T2-weighted magnetic resonance image following a remote C6–C7 spinal cord injury with heterogeneous T2 signal surrounding the spinal cord suggestive of scar tissue and cord tethering. (Adapted from Reis AJ. New surgical approach for late complications from spinal cord injury. *BMC Surgery*. 2006;6:12.)

## Treatment

### *Medical*

- Supportive treatments may include medications for neuropathic pain and spasticity

### *Exercises*

- Strengthening exercises

### *Modalities*

- Heat, cold, ultrasound, and transcutaneous electrical nerve stimulation have been used for symptomatic relief of pain and muscle spasms.

### *Injection*

- None

### *Surgical*

- Surgical treatment is considered for new or worsening symptoms.
- Preoperative percutaneous endoscopy
- Patients are kept prone postoperatively for 2 to 5 days and are only allowed to walk if there is no CSF leak demonstrated on CT imaging.

### *Consults*

- Neurologic surgery
- Physical medicine and rehabilitation

### *Complications of treatment*

- Complications related to surgery include hemorrhage, CSF leak, headache, postoperative wound infection, pseudomeningocele

## Prognosis

- Clinical improvement outcomes for pain, sensorimotor dysfunction, and bowel and bladder dysfunction range from 10% to 100%.
- Recovery of bladder function may occur with a short duration of symptoms
- Possible need for repeat detethering surgery in 3% to 16% of cases from several small studies

## Helpful Hints

- Detethering surgery or myelomeningocele repair in children results in extensive arachnoidal adhesions, causing variable adult outcomes.

## Suggested Reading

Kabayel DD, Ozdemir F, Unlu E, Bilgili N, Murat S. The effects of medical treatment and rehabilitation in a patient with adult tethered cord syndrome in the late postoperative period. *Med Sci Monit*. 2007;13(12):CS141–CS144.

# Transverse Myelitis

## Description

Transverse myelitis is an inflammatory process that affects the spinal cord.

## Etiology/Types

- Most commonly idiopathic
- Associated with connective tissue diseases and central nervous system infections

## Epidemiology

- All age groups can be affected, with peaks at ages 10 to 19 years and 30 to 39 years.
- 1,400 new cases are diagnosed per year in the United States.

## Pathogenesis

- Possible postinfectious autoimmune process due to similar epitopes between the infectious agent and spinal cord antigen (eg, tuberculosis, coxsackie virus, hepatitis B vaccination)
- May also be caused by lymphocytic activation by microbial superantigens
- Perivascular monocytic and lymphocytic infiltration
- Demyelination is prominent in the white matter tracts.
- Axonal injury

## Risk Factors

- Behçet's disease
- Herpes virus
- HIV/human T-cell leukemia/lymphoma virus-1
- Lyme disease
- Often follows respiratory, gastrointestinal, or systemic illness
- Sarcoidosis
- Sjogren's syndrome
- Syphilis
- Systemic lupus erythematosus
- 30% of pediatric cases have a history of immunization within the past month.

## Clinical Features

- Motor, sensory, and autonomic dysfunction
- Can be a presenting feature of multiple sclerosis
- Rapidly progressive paralysis over minutes, hours, or days
- Pain located at the back, abdomen, and extremities.
- Bowel and bladder dysfunction

## Natural History

- Rapidly progressive paralysis over minutes, hours, or days
- About 50% of patients become paraplegic
- Bowel and bladder dysfunction
- Numbness
- Paresthesias/dysesthesias
- Symptoms usually stop progressing after about 2 to 3 weeks.
- Persistent severe disability

## Diagnosis

### *Differential diagnosis*

- Arteriovenous malformation
- Guillain-Barré syndrome
- Ischemia
- Multiple sclerosis
- Vasculitis
- Viral myelitis

### *History*

- Determine time course and extent of neurologic deficits
- Assess for prior history of recent infection, vaccination, trauma, systemic inflammatory disease, ischemia, radiation exposure, neoplasm, or multiple sclerosis
- Bowel, bladder, and sexual dysfunction

### *Exam*

- Assess motor, sensory, reflex changes
- Assess level of spinal cord injury

### *Testing*

- Diagnosis is confirmed by CSF pleocytosis, elevated CSF IgG index, or enhancement of the spinal cord with contrast-enhanced MRI.
- MRI usually notes increased T2-weighted signal within the spinal cord and about 74% of patients demonstrate contrast enhancement.

### *Pitfalls*

- MRI may be negative in up to 40% of cases.

## Red Flags

- Rapidly progressive neurologic changes
- Bowel or bladder dysfunction

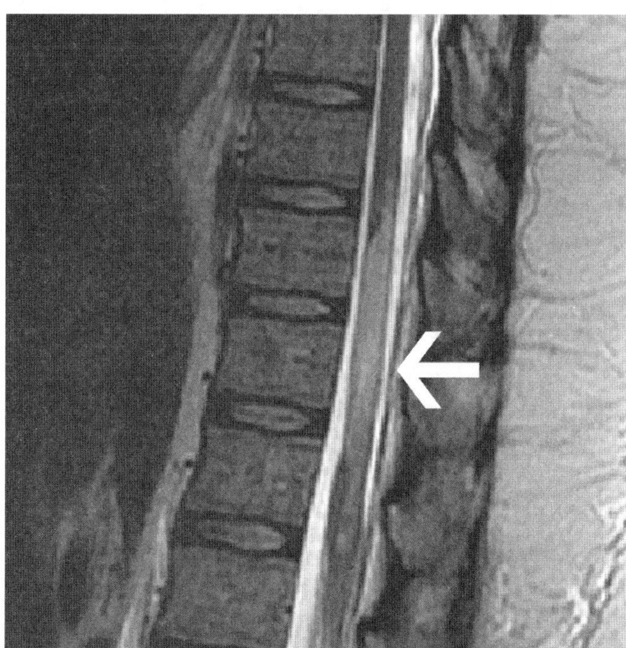

Sagittal thoracic T2-weighted magnetic resonance image demonstrating increased spinal cord signal spanning several levels (arrow) consistent with acute transverse myelitis. (Adapted from Fast A, Goldsher D. *Navigating the Adult Spine: Bridging Clinical Practice and Neuroradiology.* New York: Demos Medical Publishing, 2007:70.)

## Treatment

### Medical

- A 5-day course of intravenous methylprednisolone 1,000 mg per day followed by an oral steroid taper may improve motor recovery.
- Plasma exchange may be considered in patients who do not respond to intravenous steroids.
- Intravenous cyclophosphamide
- Bowel and bladder retraining
- Sexual dysfunction training

### Exercises

- Occupational therapy for activities of daily living
- Stretching to prevent soft tissue contractures during the acute phase
- Strengthening program
- Aerobic conditioning

### Modalities

- None

### Injection

- None

### Surgical

- None

### Consults

- Physical medicine and rehabilitation
- Neurology

### Complications of treatment

- Variable, based on the severity of the neurologic deficits

## Prognosis

- One-third of patients recover completely, one-third have permanent moderate disability, one-third have severe disability.
- Recurrent disease may occur.
- Most patients recover neurologically within 6 months but recovery can continue for 2 years.
- Poor outcome is associated with back pain, rapid progression of symptoms, cervical sensory changes, and spinal shock.
- Interleukin-6 in the CSF strongly correlates with eventual disability.

## Helpful Hints

- Depression often accompanies transverse myelitis.

## Suggested Reading

Krishnan C, Kaplin AI, Pardo CA, Kerr DA, Keswani SC. Demyelinating disorders: update on transverse myelitis. *Curr Neurol Neurosci Rep.* 2006;6(3):236–243.

# Whiplash-Associated Disorders

## Description

Whiplash-associated disorders are caused by forceful acceleration-deceleration forces in the neck resulting from rear-end or side impact, most commonly due to motor vehicle accidents.

## Etiology/Types

- Quebec Task Force Classification
  - Grade 1: neck complaints including pain, stiffness, or tenderness, without physical signs
  - Grade 2: neck complaints and musculoskeletal signs including point tenderness and decreased cervical range of motion
  - Grade 3: neck complaints and neurologic signs including upper-extremity paresthesias, muscle fatigue, a sense of heaviness
  - Grade 4: neck complaints with fracture or dislocation

## Epidemiology

- Based on insurance claims, the incidence ranges from 0.1% to 14.5% per 1,000 population
- Affects 20% to 83% of patients involved in motor vehicle collisions
- Common cause of chronic disability

## Pathogenesis

- Controversial
- Generally thought to be related to cervical sprain or strain
- Forward acceleration of the trunk and shoulders during a rear-end collision causes the cervical spine to assume an S-shaped curve with the upper cervical spine in flexion and the lower cervical spine in extension followed by neck flexion.
- Can result in tears of the ligamentum flavum, anterior longitudinal ligament, and capsular ligaments; disruption of the annulus of the intervertebral disc; fractures of the zygapophyseal (facet) joints, articular pillar, endplates, and vertebral bodies.
- Muscles do no have time to react to the sudden force.
- Strain or tear of the sternocleidomastoid, scalene, or longus colli muscles
- Longus colli muscle tears may also cause injury to the sympathetic trunk, resulting in Horner's syndrome, dizziness, and nausea.
- Temporomandibular dysfunction is related to forceful rapid jaw opening with neck extension stretching the capsule and disrupting the disc.

## Risk Factors

- Spondylosis

## Clinical Features

- Primarily a clinical diagnosis
- Delayed onset of symptoms up to 12 to 14 hours later, following the inciting event
- Neck pain at rest or with movement
- Neck stiffness
- Headache is the second most common symptom.
- Upper-extremity pain and paresthesias
- Jaw pain
- Visual changes caused by increased sympathetic tone
- Dizziness due to vestibular dysfunction or injury
- Memory and concentration dysfunction
- Psychological distress

## Natural History

- Pain generally resolve within 12 weeks, although up to 39.6% of patients may have pain for as long as 7 years.

## Diagnosis

### Differential diagnosis

- Cervical fracture or dislocation or both
- Cervical radiculopathy
- Occipital neuralgia

### History

- Delayed onset of symptoms, up to 12 to 14 hours following the inciting event
- Neck pain at rest or with movement
- Neck stiffness
- Headache is the second most common symptom.

### Exam

- Decreased cervical range of motion in all planes, mostly affecting flexion and extension

### Testing

- Imaging can be used to rule out fractures and ligament or disc injuries.
- Lateral flexion–extension X-rays may demonstrate loss of the normal lordosis and kyphotic angle, which

is thought to be due to a hypermobile segment adjacent to a hypomobile segment that results from muscle spasm.

### *Pitfalls*

- Clinical diagnosis based on symptoms and mechanism of injury

## Red Flags

- Cervical fracture or dislocation or both

## Treatment

### *Medical*

- Early mobilization may improve outcome.
- Immobilization and rest are not recommended.
- NSAIDs
- Muscle relaxants
- Mild analgesics
- Intravenous methylprednisolone
- Driving should be avoided during the acute stage.

### *Exercises*

- Cervical range of motion exercises

### *Modalities*

- Heat, cold, ultrasound, and transcutaneous electrical nerve stimulation have been used for symptomatic relief of pain and muscle spasms.
- Traction

### *Injection*

- Medial branch blocks and percutaneous radiofrequency neurotomy of the medial branches of C2–C3 or below have been found to be helpful for up to 1 year.

### *Surgical*

- Considered in the treatment of fracture or dislocation or both

### *Consults*

- Physical medicine and rehabilitation
- Neurologic and orthopedic-spine surgery

### *Complications of treatment*

- Persistent disabling pain
- Disability

## Prognosis

- Pain generally resolve within 12 weeks.
- 50% of adults report neck pain 1 year following the injury.
- 39.6% of patients may have pain as long as seven years.
- Slower recovery in patients with greater symptom severity
- Poor recovery related to postinjury psychological distress, passive coping strategies
- Prolonged worker's compensation found to be related to the severity of the collision, lack of seat belt use, nonrear-end impact, riding in a vehicle other than a car or taxi, female gender, older age, and number of dependents
- 14% to 42% of patients will develop chronic neck pain.

## Helpful Hints

- Important to rule out fracture
- Attempt to search for a possible specific diagnosis while treating the associated disorders

## Suggested Reading

Rodriquez AA, Barr KP, Burns SP. Whiplash: pathophysiology, diagnosis, treatment, and prognosis. *Muscle Nerve.* 2004;29(6):768–781.

# Zygapophyseal (Facet) Joint Pain, Cervical

## Description

Cervical zygapophyseal (facet) joint pain is due to a non-inflammatory degenerative joint disease that is characterized by progressive joint stiffness, decreased range of motion, and pain.

## Etiology/Types

- Multifactorial type includes genetic, biochemical, and biomechanical factors
- Traumatic type includes fracture, dislocation, and whiplash injuries.
- Degenerative type includes osteoarthritis.

## Epidemiology

- X-ray findings are nearly universal in individuals aged 65 years and older.
- Severity increases with advancing age.
- Prevalence estimates range from 25% to 63%.

## Pathogenesis

- Zygapophyseal (facet) joints are diarthrodial joints that are made of a fibrous capsule lined with a synovial membrane containing articular cartilage and menisci.
- C0–C1 and C1–C2 are innervated by cervical ventral rami.
- C2–C3 is innervated by two different branches of the C3 dorsal ramus.
- C3–C4 to C8–T1 are innervated by the medial branches of the cervical dorsal rami, above and below the joint.
- Not exclusively a disorder of articular cartilage but includes periarticular bone, synovial lining, and adjacent connective tissue.

## Risk Factors

- Heredity
- Increasing age, although not universal
- Joint instability or malalignment
- Neck hyperextension injury
- Trauma

## Clinical Features

- Axial neck pain with radiation from the suboccipital region to the shoulders or midback
- There are no history or physical examination findings that are specific for zygapophyseal (facet) joint pain.

## Natural History

- Unknown

## Diagnosis

### *Differential diagnosis*

- Cervical discogenic pain
- Cervical spinal stenosis
- Fibromyalgia
- Muscle strain or sprain
- Myofascial pain syndrome
- Neuralgic amyotrophy
- Occipital neuralgia
- Shoulder pathology
- Spinal cord injury
- Syringomyelia
- Thoracic outlet syndrome

### *History*

- Axial neck pain with radiation from the suboccipital region to the shoulders or midback

### *Exam*

- There are no physical examination findings that are specific for zygapophyseal (facet) joint pain.
- Possibly worsens with neck motion in a certain plane
- Decreased neck range of motion

### *Testing*

- X-rays are useful to screen for instability, fractures, and osteoarthritis
- Flexion–extension X-rays are used to assess for instability.
- MRI has demonstrated degenerative joints in up to 75% of asymptomatic adults in the seventh decade of life.
- SPECT may be useful.
- Small fractures may be present that are not detected with advanced imaging.

### *Pitfalls*

- Results of imaging need to be correlated with the patient's presenting history and physical examination.

## Red Flags

- Neurologic dysfunction

## Treatment

### Medical
- NSAIDs
- Analgesics

### Exercises
- Cervical range of motion
- Traction

### Modalities
- Heat, cold, ultrasound, and transcutaneous electrical nerve stimulation have been used for symptomatic relief of pain and muscle spasms.
- Spinal manipulation and mobilization

### Injection
- Fluoroscopically guided cervical zygapophyseal (facet) intra-articular block or medial branch block
- Radiofrequency neurotomy of the medial branches of the dorsal rami has been shown to decrease pain from several months to 1 year.
- Pulsed radiofrequency of the medial branches of the dorsal rami has demonstrated improvement up to 4 months in several small studies.

### Surgical
- Cervical fusion

### Consults
- Physical medicine and rehabilitation
- Neurologic or orthopedic-spine surgery

### Complications of treatment
- Complications related to interventional procedures
- Complications related to surgery

## Prognosis
- Unknown

## Helpful Hints
- There are no history or physical examination findings that are specific for zygapophyseal (facet) joint pain.
- Results of imaging need to be correlated with the presenting history and physical examination.

## Suggested Reading
Kirpalani D, Mitra R. Cervical facet joint dysfunction: a review. *Arch Phys Med Rehabil.* 2008;89(4):770–774.

# Zygapophyseal (Facet) Joint Pain, Lumbar

## Description

Zygapophyseal (facet) joint pain is due to a noninflammatory degenerative joint disease that is characterized by progressive joint stiffness, decreased range of motion, and pain resulting in loss of mobility.

## Etiology/Types

- Multifactorial etiology
- Genetic factors
- Biochemical factors
- Repetitive strain and low-grade trauma

## Epidemiology

- Most common at the L5–S1 level followed by the L4–L5 and L3–L4 levels
- Prevalence of zygapophyseal (facet) joint pain ranges from 15% in the younger population to 54% in the elderly population.
- Zygapophyseal (facet) joint arthrosis usually begins in the third decade of life.
- Radiographic findings are nearly universal in individuals aged 65 years and older.
- More common in males compared with females

## Pathogenesis

- Not exclusively a disorder of articular cartilage but also includes periarticular bone, synovial lining, adjacent connective tissue.
- Can be associated with disc degeneration
- 16% of the axial compressive force passes through the joints with standing and 0% occurs with sitting.
- With increased intervertebral disc herniation there is an increased axial loading of the zygapophyseal (facet) joints.
- Several studies demonstrate correlation between tropism and degenerative disc disease.
- Capsular irritation can result in reflexive spasm of the erector spinae and multifidus muscles.

## Risk Factors

- Heredity
- Increasing age, although not universal
- Intervertebral disc degeneration
- Muscle weakness
- Peripheral neuropathy
- Recurrent rotational strains
- Three-joint unit instability or malalignment

## Clinical Features

- Symptoms range from asymptomatic to severe pain in the lower back and legs with difficulty walking.
- Morning stiffness
- Pain exacerbated with lumbar extension and/or ipsilateral rotation or descending stairs.
- Pain improved with flexion
- Postural changes include age-related loss of lumbar lordosis that offloads the degenerative zygapophyseal (facet) joints.
- Referred pain associated with lower lumbar zygapophyseal (facet) joints usually extends into the lower lateral leg and occasionally to the foot.

## Natural History

- Increased risk of joint changes and pain with increasing age, although not universal
- Back pain is less common in former athletes compared with controls even in the presence of spondylosis.

## Diagnosis

### *Differential diagnosis*

- Acute or chronic infection
- Ankylosing spondylitis
- Degenerative disc disease
- Reactive arthritis
- Rheumatoid arthritis
- Trauma

### *History*

- Research has not demonstrated a reliable clinical feature that correlates with zygapophyseal (facet) joint pain.
- Dull aching pain
- Pain generally thought to improve with flexion and worsen with extension and/or rotation, or with descending stairs.

### *Exam*

- Generally believed that pain is exacerbated with lumbar extension and/or ipsilateral rotation.
- Lumbar paraspinal tenderness may be present, particularly in the sacral sulcus.

### *Testing*

- Lumbar X-rays may demonstrate loss of disc height and zygapophyseal (facet) joint sclerosis and degeneration.

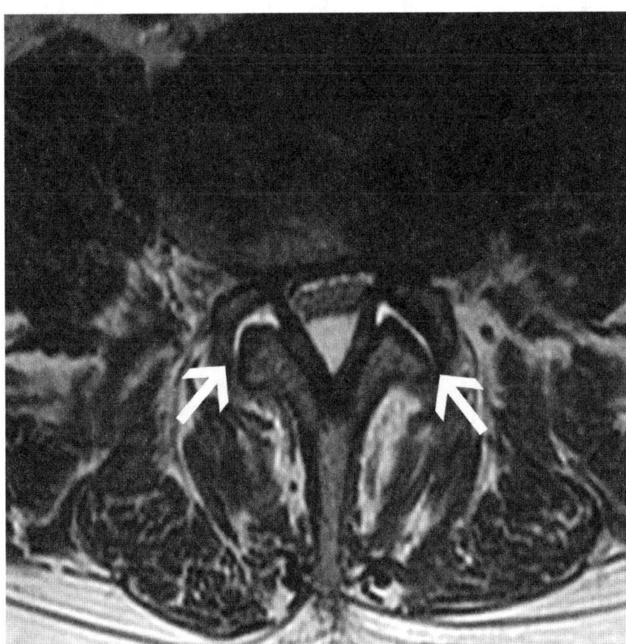

Axial lumbar T2-weighted magnetic resonance image demonstrating increased signal within the zygapophyseal joints (arrows) suggestive of an inflammatory reaction.

- Bone scan demonstrates increased uptake in regions of joint subchondral sclerosis.
- MRI may demonstrate thickened, irregular zygapophyseal (facet) joints with increased T2-weighted fluid signal within the joint space.
- Fluoroscopically guided anesthetic blockade of the suspected zygapophyseal (facet) joint or the corresponding medial branches is the most reliable test for identifying the specific zygapophyseal (facet) associated with the pain, but the false positive rate ranges from 25% to 41%.

### *Pitfalls*
- A distended joint capsule may compress a nerve root or the spinal cord.
- Considerable overlap of pain referral patterns

## Red Flags
- Progressive neurologic dysfunction

## Treatment

### *Medical*
- NSAIDs
- Analgesics
- Transdermal anesthetic and anti-inflammatory patches in the older population

### *Exercises*
- General strengthening and stretching exercises
- Yoga

### *Modalities*
- Heat, cold, ultrasound, and transcutaneous electrical nerve stimulation have been used for symptomatic relief of pain and muscle spasms.
- Spinal manipulation and mobilization

### *Injection*
- Fluoroscopically guided radiofrequency denervation of the medial branches of the target zygapophyseal (facet) joint
- Fluoroscopically guided intra-articular joint steroid and local anesthetic injections

### *Surgical*
- Lumbar fusion

### *Consults*
- Physical medicine and rehabilitation
- Neurologic or orthopedic-spine surgery

### *Complications of treatment*
- Complications related to surgery include infection and bleeding, general anesthesia risks.
- Complications related to the interventional procedures include neuritis in up to 5% of patients.

## Prognosis
- Radiofrequency denervation has been shown to provide up to 1 year of relief with anecdotal reports of longer duration in select patients
- Surgery has been shown to result in improvement in select patients.

## Helpful Hints
- Beware of considerable overlap of pain referral patterns.

## Suggested Reading
Cohen SP, Raja SN. Pathogenesis, diagnosis, and treatment of lumbar zygapophyseal (facet) joint pain. *Anesthesiology.* 2007;106(3):591–614.

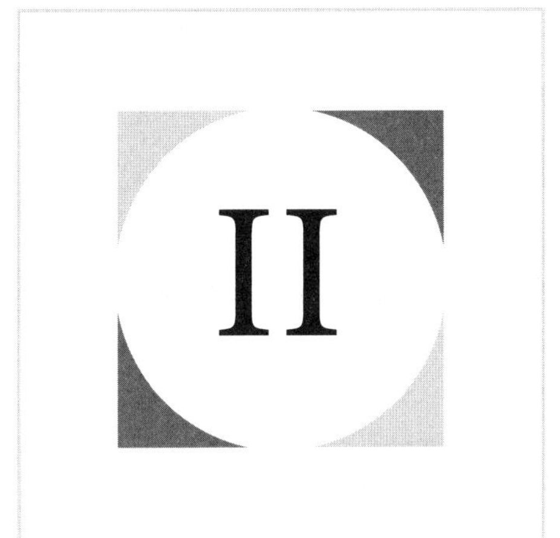


# Spine-Mimicking Conditions

# Carpal Tunnel Syndrome

## Description

Carpal tunnel syndrome caused by compression of the median nerve within the carpal tunnel is the most common focal compression neuropathy of the upper extremity.

## Etiology/Types

- Compression of the median nerve as it passes through the carpal tunnel, due to swelling of the flexor tendon lining, fracture, joint dislocation, or inflammatory arthritis

## Epidemiology

- Lifetime risk of 10%
- Female to male ratio 3:1
- Neck pain in those with median nerve sensory abnormalities is 24%.

## Pathogenesis

- Compression of the median nerve due to a variety of factors results in loss of motor and sensory function along the distribution of the median nerve in the hand.

## Risk Factors

- Amyloidosis
- Awkward wrist positioning
- Diabetes
- Edema
- Gout or pseudogout
- Hypo- or hyperthyroidism
- Lyme disease
- Most cases not work related
- Obesity
- Pregnancy
- Repetitive hand motions
- Septic arthritis

## Clinical Features

- Numbness or paresthesias of the palmar side of the radial three and one-half digits
- Thenar atrophy with severe disease
- Loss of dexterity
- Inability to pick up or manipulate small objects
- Dull aching discomfort in the forearm or upper arm may occur in up to 45% of patients and is associated with milder median nerve entrapment at the wrist and greater hand paresthesias.
- 84% of confirmed cases have nocturnal hand paresthesias.
- 82% have paresthesias aggravated by activities of the hand.

## Natural History

- Progressive pain followed by increasing numbness, tingling and/or weakness of the median nerve innervated sensory, and motor distribution
- Pain eventually subsides as neurologic deficits worsen.
- Wasting of the thenar muscles results in a "simian hand" and loss of the ability to oppose the thumb to the little finger.
- Loss of manual dexterity with disease progression

## Diagnosis

### *Differential diagnosis*

- Anterior interosseous nerve syndrome
- C6 or C7 radiculopathy
- Pronator syndrome
- Supracondylar process syndrome

### *History*

- Numbness or paresthesias of the palmar side of the radial three and one-half digits, hand, and wrist
- Pain may radiate distally into the hand or proximally up the arm.
- Progressive tingling during the day
- Pain worse in the evening
- "Flick" sign is often described by patients who "flick" their wrist to relieve symptoms.

### *Exam*

- Tinel's test is positive if tingling is reproduced with tapping of the median nerve at the wrist from proximal to distal; 87% specificity.
- Phalen's test or the reverse Phalen's test reproduces a patient's pain with wrist flexion or extension to 90 degrees, respectively at 60 seconds; 60% specificity.
- Durkin's compression test is positive if symptoms are reproduced with direct compression of the carpal tunnel.
- Weak thumb abduction is rare.
- Thenar atrophy is rare.
- Loss of sensation over the median distribution

### Testing

- Electrodiagnostic testing is used to diagnose, assess severity, and to rule out cervical radiculopathy, plexopathy, and peripheral neuropathy.
- Normal electrodiagnostic studies may be found in up to 8% of patients with symptoms.
- MRI is used to assess for cysts, tenosynovitis, and aberrant muscles.

### Pitfalls

- Pregnancy-related symptoms usually resolve following delivery.

## Red Flags

- Severe weakness or numbness
- "Simian hand"

## Treatment

### Medical

- Education to avoid repetitive wrist and hand movements
- Wrist splints at a neutral angle are most effective when used within 3 months of symptom onset.
- Wrist splints only at night are not as effective as full-time use.
- Short-term NSAIDs
- Oral prednisone may be helpful in the short term.

### Exercises

- Nerve and tendon gliding exercises
- Strengthening and stretching

### Modalities

- Ultrasound

### Injection

- Steroid injection into the carpal tunnel may provide temporary relief.

### Surgical

- Open or endoscopic surgical release of the transverse carpal tunnel ligament is considered in patients with severe nerve entrapment who have not responded to conservative treatment.

### Consults

- Physical medicine and rehabilitation
- Orthopedic hand surgery
- Plastic surgery

### Complications of treatment

- Surgical complications include nerve or arterial injury, hypertrophic scarring, tendon damage, stiffness, post-operative infection, hematoma

## Prognosis

- Symptoms recur in about 80% of patients after 1 year with conservative treatment.
- A 2-year follow up of untreated carpal tunnel syndrome noted that 67% of patients remained the same electrodiagnostically with almost 8% deteriorating and 25% improving.

## Helpful Hints

- Carpal tunnel syndrome is a clinical diagnosis with electrodiagnostic confirmation.

## Suggested Reading

Chow CS, Hung LK, Chiu CP, et al. Is symptomatology useful in distinguishing between carpal tunnel syndrome and cervical spondylosis? *Hand Surg.* 2005;10(1):1–5.

# Complex Regional Pain Syndrome (Reflex Sympathetic Dystrophy)

## Description

Complex regional pain syndrome is a chronic pain syndrome that often develops with or without an inciting event, is more severe than the original injury, and leads to pain and functional loss of the affected extremity and eventual impairment.

## Etiology/Types

- Thought to be caused by the sympathetic nervous system or an immune response
- 14% to 46% report a minor fracture.
- 10% to 29% report a sprain or strain.
- 3% to 24% occurs postsurgery.
- 2% to 25% report no inciting event.
- Reported in up to 61% of poststroke patients
- International Association for the Study of Pain (IASP) classification type 1 reflex sympathetic dystrophy (RSD)
  - Syndrome that develops following a noxious event, the severity or which is disproportionate to the inciting event.
  - No nerve lesion
  - Symptoms may not be isolated to the affected nerve distribution.
  - The affected area may demonstrate changes in cutaneous blood flow, sudomotor activity, edema, and hyperalgesia or allodynia.
  - More common than type 2.
  - Often mild presentation
- IASP classification of type 2
  - Causalgia, allodynia or hyperpathia after major trauma and/or major nerve injury
  - May not be isolated to the affected nerve distribution
  - The affected area may demonstrate changes in cutaneous blood flow, sudomotor activity, edema, and hyperalgesia or allodynia.
  - Often affects the hand or foot.
  - Often severe presentation

## Epidemiology

- Incidence is greater than 26 per 100,000.
- Most common in older women with an upper limb fracture
- Mean age range from 36 to 46 years
- Female predominance

## Pathogenesis

- Sensitization of primary nociceptor afferents results in the release of inflammatory mediators
- Sensitization of the sympathetic nervous system
- Pseudoinflammatory

## Risk Factors

- Immobilization
- Increased risk with human leukocyte antigen-DQ1, DR13, and DR2
- Limb trauma such as ankle sprain, scaphoid fracture, crush injury, or following surgery
- Type 2 is more common with brachial plexus avulsions.
- Psychological predisposition

## Clinical Features

- Erythematous or cyanosed blotchy skin
- Skin atrophy
- Skin edema occurs in up to 81% of patients
- Loss of normal skin creases
- Reduced or excessive sweating
- Increased or decreased temperature
- Excess or loss of hair
- Nail ridges, clubbing, curve, or brittleness
- Restricted passive range of motion, contractures
- Osteoporosis
- Muscle wasting and weakness with up to 78% reporting greatly decreased grip strength
- Myoclonic jerks, spasms, dystonia, tremor
- Urinary sphincter or detruser dysfunction
- Allodynia—normal sensory stimuli causing pain

## Natural History

- Stage 1: early acute stage characterized by pain and sensory dysfunction, vasomotor and sudomotor dysfunction, and edema
- Stage 2 (dystrophic stage): occurs within 3–6 months and is characterized by increased pain and sensory and vasomotor dysfunction, as well as motor and trophic changes
- Stage 3 (atrophic stage): characterized by decreased pain and sensory dysfunction with continued vasomotor dysfunction with increased motor and trophic changes
- Loss of limb function

## Diagnosis

### Differential diagnosis

- Fracture
- Neuropathy/neuropathic pain
- Radiculopathy

### History

- Usually spontaneous and severe burning pain
- Variable weakness or muscle wasting
- Involuntary movements
- Predominately in the distal extremity
- Hypo- or hyperalgesia and allodynia

### Exam

- 74% of patients present with allodynia.
- 70% report decreased joint range of motion.
- 66% report skin color asymmetry.
- 56% report skin temperature asymmetry.
- 56% report weakness.
- 14% report dystonia.
- 9% report tremor.

### Testing

- Is used to rule out other disorders
- X-rays may demonstrate spotty osteoporotic changes in the affected limb.
- Bone scan may demonstrate increased uptake indicating increased bone metabolism.
- Electrodiagnostic studies can be used to rule out neurologic causes.

### Pitfalls

- Unpredictable course

## Red Flags

- Loss of limb function
- Severe pain

## Treatment

### Medical

- Immobilization for as short a time as possible.
- Trial of gabapentin, tricyclic antidepressants, duloxetine, opioids, bisphosphonates, prednisone, vitamin C
- Psychological evaluation in patients with two or more months of symptoms
- Remove aggravating factors

### Exercises

- Joint range of motion
- Stress loading of the limb
- Coordination/dexterity
- Aquatic therapy

### Modalities

- Compression devices for edema management
- Contrast bath for desensitization
- Transcutaneous electrical nerve stimulation

### Injection

- Sympathetic block
- Intravenous regional block

### Surgical

- Intrathecal baclofen
- Spinal cord stimulator

### Consults

- Pain management

### Complications of treatment

- Variable

## Prognosis

- May resolve within weeks or continue for years
- Only 29% of patients become pain free.
- Severe impairments in up to 64% of patients

## Helpful Hints

- Important to identify and treat earlier in the course of the disease
- Surgery may worsen symptoms.

## Suggested Reading

Atkins RM. Complex regional pain syndrome. *J Bone Joint Surg Br.* 2003;85(8):1100–1106.

# Fibromyalgia

## Description

Fibromyalgia is an idiopathic, chronic, nonarticular, soft tissue pain syndrome with widespread musculoskeletal pain and generalized tender points.

## Etiology/Types

- Unknown genetic and environmental factors
- Possible role for polymorphisms of genes in the serotoninergic, dopaminergic, and catecholaminergic systems

## Epidemiology

- Underdiagnosed
- Prevalence is reported to be 3.4% in females and 0.5% in males.
- Most commonly affects women 20 to 50 years of age.
  - Also described in males, adolescents, and children

## Pathogenesis

- Part of a spectrum of diseases called central sensitization syndromes, characterized by systemic symptoms including muscle pain
- Other central sensitization syndromes commonly associated with fibromyalgia include irritable bowel syndrome, irritable bladder, dysmenorrhea, premenstrual syndrome, restless leg syndrome, and temporomandibular joint pain

## Risk Factors

- Anxiety
- Depression
- Epstein–Barr virus
- Lyme disease
- Parvovirus
- Peripheral pain syndrome
- Physical trauma
- Predisposing social characteristics include divorce, failure to complete high school, and low income.
- Q fever
- Somatization disorder

## Clinical Features

- Diagnosis is based on the American College of Rheumatology 1990 criteria, although a number of physicians have been critical of its usefulness as the original criteria was formed as part of a research protocol.
  - Bilateral widespread pain above and below the waist including the axial spine for at least 3 months
  - Presence of 11 tender points among the nine pairs of specified sites (18 points). Using moderate and consistent pressure of the dominant thumb [8.8 lbs (4.0 kg)], which should begin to blanch the examiner's thumbnail
- Sleep disturbance
- Cognitive difficulties
- Fatigue
- Headache
- Morning stiffness
- Paresthesias
- Anxiety

## Natural History

- Progressive pain occasionally associated with disability

## Diagnosis

### Differential diagnosis

- Chronic fatigue syndrome
- Conversion disorder
- Hypothyroidism
- Metabolic or inflammatory myopathies
- Myofascial pain syndrome
- Polymyalgia rheumatica

### History

- Pain at multiple sites
- Low back pain
- Neck pain
- Stiffness, burning, or soreness that improves throughout the day
- Subjective swollen joints or paresthesias without objective findings
- Worsened by cold or humid weather, poor sleep, and physical or mental stress
- Improved with warm and dry weather, moderate physical activity, relaxation, and proper sleep

### Exam

- Decreased activity may manifest as weakness on motor testing and decreased coordination and endurance

### Testing

- Used to rule out other diagnoses

### Pitfalls

- Should not be a diagnosis of exclusion

## Red Flags

- Severe pain

## Treatment

### Medical

- Antidepressant medications such as amitriptyline or selective serotonin reuptake inhibitors
- Ultram
- Cyclobenzaprine
- Pregabalin
- NSAIDs
- Analgesics
- Cognitive behavioral therapy is used to help patients understand the effect of thoughts, expectations, and beliefs on symptoms.
- Patient education through lectures, handouts, or group meetings
- Proper sleep hygiene

### Exercises

- General strengthening, stretching, and conditioning program
- The type of exercise is not important as much as maintaining the exercise regimen.
- Improvement may be related to endogenous opioid production or by increasing resistance to microtrauma related to daily activity.

### Modalities

- Heat, cold, ultrasound, and transcutaneous electrical nerve stimulation have been used for symptomatic relief of pain and muscle spasms.

### Injection

- Trigger point injections for symptoms of myofascial pain

### Surgical

- None

### Consults

- Rheumatology
- Physical medicine and rehabilitation
- Psychiatry or psychology to address anxiety, depression, and kinesiophobia
- Vocational rehabilitation

### Complications of treatment

- Variable

## Prognosis

- Currently there is no treatment but patients may be able to lead normal functional lives with treatment.

## Helpful Hints

- Important to address the psychological impact of the disease as well as the physical impact

## Suggested Readings

Clauw DJ. Fibromyalgia: update on mechanisms and management. *J Clin Rheumatol.* 2007;13(2):102–109.

Harden RN. Muscle pain syndromes. *Am J Phys Med Rehabil.* 2007;86(suppl l):S47–S58.

# Herpes Zoster

## Description

Herpes zoster, also known as shingles, is a latent reactivation of varicella-zoster infection (chicken pox) characterized by an erythematous, papular, and/or vesicular rash that is associated with pain in the distribution of a peripheral sensory nerve root.

## Etiology/Types

- Caused by the varicella-zoster virus (VZV), which is one of the eight herpes viruses

## Epidemiology

- More common in the elderly and in individuals with decreased immune function

## Pathogenesis

- VZV attaches to the hosts cells by binding to a heparin sulfate proteoglycan.
- The initial infection, known as chicken pox, is associated with a viremia and cutaneous eruptions.
- The VZV remains dormant in the sensory ganglion of the spinal cord.
- The virus reactivates with decreased host immunity, spreading within the cutaneous sensory neuron found within the dorsal root ganglion, and traveling centrally and peripherally within the nerve.
- Large, myelinated sensory fibers are most commonly affected.
- Inflammation and hemorrhage within the dorsal root ganglion, the posterior horn of the spinal cord. and corresponding motor neuron on the anterior horn
- VZV reactivation also scars and fibrosis the peripheral nerve.
- Patient is infectious during the reactivation period and prior to the development of vesicles.

## Risk Factors

- Advancing age
- Decreased immune activity

## Clinical Features

- 4- to 28-day prodome of nonspecific constitutional symptoms such as fever and malaise
- Pain first develops 4 to 7 days before the skin manifestations.
- Cutaneous erythema, edema, vesicular eruptions, and hemorrhage eventually develop.
- Scarring, atrophy, and macular or papular depigmentation
- 55% of cases affect the thoracic spinal nerves.

## Natural History

- Pain along a dermatome begins first, followed a week later by erythematous skin papules that coalesce into vesicles.
- The vesicles dry within days
- Immunosupressed individuals may develop transverse myelitis, encephalitis. or cerebral vasculitis with associated signs and symptoms.
- Postherpetic neuralgia occurs with continued pain following the resolution of cutaneous disease and may take 2 to 4 weeks to resolve.
- Persistent postherpetic neuralgia is reported by up to 50% of patents aged 70 years and above.
- Depression may occur due to the persistent pain.
- Visceral or autonomic nerve dysfunction

## Diagnosis

### *Differential diagnosis*

- Herpes simplex virus
- Intercostal neuralgia
- Muscle strain
- Radiculopathy
- Superficial pyoderma

### *History*

- Shooting, burning, tingling, or sharp pain with skin dysesthesias along the sensory nerve distribution
- Localized erythematous papules develop within a week, which form into vesicles following a segmental distribution, but may include up to three dermatomes.

### *Exam*

- Skin lesions begin as an erythematous region and eventually coalesce into vesicles and groups of vesicles on an erythematous base.
- Cutaneous lesions do not cross the midline.
- The vesicles crust and desquamate within 3 weeks.
- Old lesions appear as hypopigmented macules or papules.
- Motor loss, which is usually temporary, may be associated with corresponding motor neuron involvement.
- Fever and localized lymphadenopathy

### Testing

- Viral culture
- Direct immunofluorescence assay

### Pitfalls

- Dysesthetia or total sensory loss at the site of involvement

## Red Flags

- The patient may be contagious if seen prior to the development of dry crusted vesicles.

## Treatment

### Medical

- Patients with vesicles should have limited exposure to other people.
- Healthy patients younger than 50 years of age can be treated with analgesics, antipruritics, mild sedatives, topical antibiotic ointment.
- Immune-competent patients aged 50 years and older can be treated with corticosteroids, valacyclovir, or adenosine monophosphate.
- Immunocompromised patients should be treated with aggressive antiviral therapy.
- Postherpetic neuralgia can be treated with amitriptyline, gabapentin, topical capsaicin, or lidocaine patch.

### Exercises

- None

### Modalities

- Postherpetic neuralgia may be treated with a transcutaneous electrical nerve stimulator.

### Injection

- Postherpetic neuralgia may be treated with local nerve root blocks.

### Surgical

- None

### Consults

- Infectious disease
- Dermatology if the presenting signs and symptoms are atypical
- Physical medicine and rehabilitation

### Complications of treatment

- Variable

## Prognosis

- Usually self-limiting
- Most commonly results in no or minimal disability
- Older patients are more likely to demonstrate postherpetic neuralgia, which may result in significant disability.

## Helpful Hints

- Not associated with lumbar radiculopathies
- Patients are infectious prior to the development of vesicles.

## Suggested Reading

Straus SE, Ostrove JM, Inchauspé G, et al. NIH conference. Varicella-zoster virus infections. Biology, natural history, treatment, and prevention. *Ann Intern Med.* 1988;108(2):221–237.

# Hip–Spine Syndrome

## Description

Hip–spine syndrome (HSS) describes a symptom complex resulting from concurrent degenerative hip and degenerative disc disease of the lumbar spine.

## Etiology/Types

- Degenerative changes in the hip and lumbar spine increase with advancing age.
- Simple HSS: Pathology from either the hip or the spine that is clearly identified as the primary cause of pain.
- Complex HSS: Degenerative changes at the hip and spine that both contribute to the pain complaint.
- Secondary HSS: Hip and spine pathology that are interrelated due to a hip flexion, adduction deformity of the hip, or scoliosis.

## Epidemiology

- Radiographic changes associated with hip osteoarthritis are found in up to 12% of patients older than 80 years of age.
- MRI findings of spinal stenosis are found in up to 20% of asymptomatic patients over 60 years of age.

## Pathogenesis

- L4 nerve root involvement can present with weakness and wasting of the quadriceps muscles and loss of the patellar reflex.
- Synovitis of the hip may result in buttock pain that radiates to the groin and down the anterior thigh.
- A fixed flexion deformity may result with continued inflammation at the hip joint.
- A flexion deformity of the hip may rotate the pelvis forward, increasing the lumbar lordosis and resulting in increased zygapophyseal (facet) joint subluxation and foraminal narrowing.
- Scoliosis may cause pelvic tilt uncovering the ball of the femur on the socket, increasing the risk for hip joint degeneration.
- A fixed hip adduction deformity may cause pelvic obliquity, resulting in lumbar scoliosis and eventually causing nerve root involvement.

## Risk Factors

- Alterations at the L4–L5 and L5–S1 lumbar discs
- Poor posture and sagittal alignment
- Antalgic gait

## Clinical Features

- Hip pain, L3–L4 segment instability or L4 root involvement can present as pain over the anterior aspect of the thigh.
- A limp, groin pain, and limited hip internal range of motion are more predictive of a hip disorder.

## Natural History

- Progressive pain and mobility deficit

## Diagnosis

### *Differential diagnosis*

- Avascular necrosis of the hip
- Greater trochanteric bursitis
- Groin pain related to an L3 or L4 radiculopathy
- Hip osteonecrosis
- Labral tear
- Sciatica

### *History*

- Groin pain is more common with true intra-articular hip pathology.
  - Pain is exacerbated by ambulation but relieved with rest.
  - Progression to continued pain at night
- Buttock and back pain can be difficult to differentiate.

### *Exam*

- The goal is to isolate the hip joint and lower lumbar region while attempting to reproduce the characteristic pain.
- A femoral nerve stretch with hip hyperextension while the patient is prone can reproduce the characteristic pain of an L4 radiculopathy.
- Ely's test involves having the patient prone, fully flexing the knee, pushing the heel toward the buttock.
  - Stretching of the rectus femoris will cause the hip to flex, causing the buttocks to rise.
- There may be wasting of the quadriceps muscle.
- Pain may be reproduced with hip flexion or internal rotation.
- Limited internal hip range of motion
- Antalgic gait
- Often physical exam findings are difficult to differentiate from age-expected changes.
- Straight leg raise to assess for radiculopathy

### Testing

- X-rays may demonstrate hip joint osteoarthritis.
- MRI is useful in assessing hip joint pathology, labral tears, or fracture as well as axial spine pathology.
- CT may be used to assess for joint pathology or fracture.

### Pitfalls

- Improper diagnosis

## Red Flags

- Severe quadriceps muscle wasting
- Severe weakness, numbness, or tingling in the lower extremities
- Bowel or bladder changes

## Treatment

### Medical

- NSAIDs and analgesics

### Exercises

- Myofascial release of the hip flexor contracture
- Pelvic alignment and stability
- Lower-extremity strengthening and stretching

### Modalities

- Heat, cold, ultrasound, and transcutaneous electrical nerve stimulation have been used for symptomatic relief of pain and muscle spasms.

### Injection

- Trigger point release of the iliopsoas muscle
- Fluoroscopically guided or ultrasound-guided hip anesthetic block can be used assess hip joint involvement.
- Fluoroscopically guided, contrast-enhanced L3 or L4 nerve root block is used to assess its contribution to hip pain.

### Surgical

- A hip osteotomy or total hip arthroplasty may correct the hyperlordosis, possibly relieving lower back pain, although it has not been demonstrated to change spinal sagittal radiographic angles.
- With severe spinal stenosis, lumbar decompression should be considered first.

### Consults

- Physical medicine and rehabilitation
- Neurologic or orthopedic-spine surgery

### Complications of treatment

- Lumbar decompression for patients with spine disorders will not alleviate the pain associated with a hip arthrosis.
- Foot drop following hip arthroplasty can occur in patients with severe spinal stenosis; thought to be related to a double-crush nerve injury.

## Prognosis

- Good for patients in whom the underlying pathology is identified.

## Helpful Hints

- Always screen the hip and lumbar spine to help with possible differentiation in all patients with either complaint.

## Suggested Reading

Ben-Galim P, Ben-Galim T, Rand N, et al. Hip-spine syndrome: the effect of total hip replacement surgery on low back pain in severe osteoarthritis of the hip. *Spine.* 2007;32(19):2099–2102.

# Lyme Disease

## Description

Lyme disease is a tick-borne infectious disease that can result in progressive rheumatologic, neurologic, and cardiac dysfunction.

## Etiology/Types

- Lyme disease is caused by the spirochete *Borrelia burgdorferi*.

## Epidemiology

- Most common vector-borne infectious disease in the United States
- 15,000 cases are reported annually.
- Most common in the Northeast and Midwest regions of the United States as well as the California and Oregon coasts.
- Endemic areas are associated with large deer populations, which carry the tick species *Ixodes*, responsible for transmitting *B. burgdorferi* to humans.

## Pathogenesis

- The *Ixodes* species of tick has a four-stage, 2-year life cycle, which includes the egg, larval, nymphal, and adult stages.
- The host of the nymph and larval stages is the white-footed mouse, which acts as a reservoir for the spirochete allowing for transmission to the tick.
- When the infected adult tick falls off the deer and attaches to the human host, it takes 24 hours for the spirochete to mobilize to the salivary glands of the tick and infect the host.
- It is thought that the spirochete remains in the body during the disease progression.

## Risk Factors

- Chronic arthritis associated with Lyme disease is more common with histocompatibility type DR4
- Outdoor activities

## Clinical Features

- Early disease is associated with erythema migrans at the site of the tick bite referred to as a target lesion.
- Local lymphadenopathy
- Flulike symptoms
- Cardiac manifestations such as various degrees of heart block may occur within 7 months.
- Neurologic manifestations such as lymphocytic meningitis, radiculitis, polyneuropathy, cranial nerve palsies, and encephalopathy may occur within weeks to 12 months.
- Polyarthritis may last from 4 days to 2 years.
- The most commonly affected joints are the knee, shoulder, hip, elbow, ankle, wrist, and temporomandibular.
- Up to 32% of patients report back and neck pain.
- Late disease manifestations include persistent skin infection called acrodermatis chronica atrophicans; progressive encephalomyelitis; late polyneuropathy; and articular arthritis.

## Natural History

- The initial stage is characterized by a general malaise similar to a flulike illness with neck and lower back pain associated with a characteristic erythema migrans.
- The later stage includes cardiac and neurologic symptoms such as polyradiculitis, arthritis, chronic fatigue, and encephalomyelitis.

## Diagnosis

### *Differential diagnosis*

- Babesiosis
- Ehrlichiosis
- Radiculopathy

### *History*

- Outdoor recreation
- Tick bite
- Flu-like symptoms
- Myalgias, arthralgias
- Skin rash

### *Exam*

- Erythema migrans
- Regional lymphadenopathy
- Musculoskeletal complaints are constant, irrespective of activity.
- Irregular pulse with cardiac manifestations
- Neurologic abnormalities include radiculitis, neurologic deficits, cranial nerve dysfunction, and impaired cognition.
- Late disease manifestations include skin atrophy, persistent arthritis, cognitive deficits, and spastic paresis.

### Testing

- Elevated erythrocyte sedimentation rate
- CSF may demonstrate increased protein concentration, lymphocytic pleocytosis, and antibodies to *B. burgdorferi.*
- Synovial fluid analysis from an affected joint demonstrates an inflammatory arthropathy.
- The enzyme-linked immunosorbent assay (ELISA) test, confirmed by Western blot analysis can be used to detect the presence of antibodies.
- X-rays may demonstrate loss of articular cartilage, osseous erosions, or chondrocalcinosis.
- MRI may demonstrate scattered white lesions similar to other demyelinating diseases.

### Pitfalls

- Missed diagnosis

## Red Flags

- Progressive neurologic changes

## Treatment

### Medical

- Children and pregnant females are treated with amoxicillin.
- Early stage treated with doxycycline or tetracycline
- Erythromycin is used with penicillin allergy.
- Antibiotics for 14 to 21 days
- In the late stage, intravenous antibiotics for 14 to 28 days are given, although the treatment response may be delayed up to 6 to 8 months.

### Exercises

- Gentle strengthening and stretching exercises

### Modalities

- Heat, cold, ultrasound, and transcutaneous electrical nerve stimulation have been used for symptomatic relief of pain and muscle spasms.

### Injection

- Possible joint fluid aspiration to rule out a septic joint

### Surgical

- None

### Consults

- Infectious disease
- Rheumatology

### Complications of treatment

- Progressive disease due to incomplete treatment

## Prognosis

- Excellent prognosis if identified early and treated with antibiotics.
- Radiculopathy and neuropathies may resolve in 24 months.
- Poor prognosis with neurologic deficits

## Helpful Hints

- Proper dress during late spring to late summer

## Suggested Reading

Feder HM Jr, Johnson BJ, O'Connell S, et al. A critical appraisal of "chronic Lyme disease." *N Engl J Med.* 2007;357(14):1422–1430.

# Peripheral Neuropathy

## Description

Peripheral neuropathy indicates damage to the peripheral nerve. Symptoms generally include weakness, numbness, burning pain, and loss of reflexes.

## Etiology/Types

- Demyelinating neuropathies
- Focal and multifocal neuropathies
- Motor and sensory neuropathies
- Small fiber and autonomic neuropathies
- Chronic axonal neuropathies
- Inheritable neuropathies
- Guillain-Barré syndrome (GBS)
- Chronic inflammatory demyelinating polyradiculopathy (CIDP)

## Epidemiology

- 2% to 8% prevalence of neuropathy that increases with age
- Diabetes mellitus: most commonly presenting as distal symmetric sensorimotor neuropathy

## Pathogenesis

- Damage to the axon results in wallerian degeneration, which leaves the surrounding stroma intact.
- Neuronopathies result in damage proximally at the dorsal root ganglion and/or motor root.
- Myelinopathies result in damage to the myelin sheath.

## Risk Factors

- Diabetes mellitus is most common.
- Environmental exposures to solvents, acrylamide, and arsenic
- Hereditary factors
- Medications include amiodarone, statins, phenytoin, chemotherapy, and antibiotics.

## Clinical Features

- The initial presentation usually includes pain, weakness, altered sensation, or autonomic symptoms.
- Advanced changes include distal muscle wasting and weakness, sensory loss in a glove-and-stocking distribution, and loss of deep tendon reflexes.
- Neuropathies marked by wallerian degeneration exhibit symmetric length-dependent changes affecting the feet followed by the hands.
- Mononeuropathies are usually due to thyroid disease, occupation, pregnancy, or amyloidosis.
- Vasculitic mononeuropathies can occur over 24 to 72 hours
- Focal symptoms may allow for the identification of the individual affected nerve or root.
- Demyelinating neuropathies usually affect the longer fibers.
- Dorsal root ganglionopathies present with multisegmental sensory changes
- Small fiber dysfunction results in autonomic symptoms, loss of temperature, and pain.

## Natural History

- Variable

## Diagnosis

### Differential diagnosis

- Cervical spondylotic myelopathy (elderly)
- Chemicals: solvents, acrylamide, and arsenic
- Myelopathy
- Pharmaceuticals: amiodarone, statins, phenytoin, chemotherapy, and antibiotics
- Recreational drugs include tobacco, alcohol, and cocaine.
- Spinal cord injury
- Spinocerebellar syndromes
- Transverse myelitis
- Vitamin $B_{12}$ deficiency

### History

- Pins and needles sensation
- Numbness
- Burning sensation
- Unsteadiness or stumbling
- Weakness/difficulty with fine motor control

### Exam

- Facial weakness: GBS
- Proximal motor weakness: GBS, CIDP
- Loss of distal reflexes: length-dependent axonopathies
- Generalized loss of reflexes: acquired demyelinating neuropathies
- Sensory testing should test large fiber (proprioception and vibration) as well as small fiber (pain, temperature and pinprick).

- Small-fiber involvement assessed via papillary light reflex and standing and supine postural blood pressure measurements.

### Testing

- Preliminary laboratory testing should include a complete blood count, fasting blood glucose levels, glucose tolerance test, renal function tests, liver function tests, thyroid function, Vitamin $B_{12}$, folate, paraprotein screen, vasculitis screen, and erythrocyte sedimentation rate.
- Electrodiagnostic studies
- Nerve biopsy considered with the possibility of a systemic disorder
- CSF analysis can be used to determine if the CSF protein is elevated with cases of CIDP.
- Anti-GM1 and anti-GD1a antibodies are found in GBS.

### Pitfalls

- Carcinoma of the prostate
- Hypokalemia
- Arteriovenous malformation
- Tumor of the conus medullaris
- Difficult differentiating residual deficits from a chronic process

## Red Flags

- Transverse myelitis
- Arteriovenous malformation
- Tumor of the conus medullaris

## Treatment

### Medical

- Diabetes management
- $B_{12}$ replacement
- CIDP: corticosteroids, intravenous immunoglobulin, plasma exchange
- Neuropathic pain: gabapentin, anticonvulsants, tricyclic antidepressants, and tramadol

### Exercises

- Generalized strengthening and stretching

### Modalities

- Heat, cold, ultrasound, and transcutaneous electrical nerve stimulation have been used for symptomatic relief of pain and muscle spasms.

### Injection

- None

### Surgical

- None

### Consults

- Physical medicine and rehabilitation
- Neurology

### Complications of treatment

- Variable

## Prognosis

- Variable, can result in severe morbidity and mortality

## Helpful Hints

- About 20% of neuropathies remain undiagnosed.

## Suggested Reading

Richardson JK. The clinical identification of peripheral neuropathy among older persons. *Arch Phys Med Rehabil.* 2002;83(11):1553–1558.

# Piriformis Syndrome (Pseudosciatica)

## Description

Piriformis syndrome is sciatica-like pain due to impingement of the sciatic nerve as it courses through the piriformis muscle.

## Etiology/Types

- Primary piriformis syndrome describes all pathology related to the piriformis muscle, such as myofascial pain.
- Secondary piriformis syndrome is reserved for buttock pain with or without radiation down the lower extremity based on the location of the pathology in relation to the structures exiting the sciatic notch.

## Epidemiology

- The incidence is thought to be 6% to 8% of all low back pain cases.
- Most often noted in the 30- to 40-year age group
- The female to male ratio is thought to be 3–6:1.

## Pathogenesis

- The piriformis muscle is the largest of the short external rotators of the hip.
- Others external rotators of the hip include the superior and inferior gemellus, quadratus femoris, and obturator internus muscles.
- The piriformis muscle originates from the second to fourth sacral vertebrae, exiting the pelvis through the sciatic notch, and inserting on the upper portion of the greater trochanter.
- Variations are known to exist in the course of the sciatic nerve through the piriformis muscle.
- The exact mechanism of sciatica remains unknown, although theories include nerve entrapment due to adhesions from an initial injury such as a fall, compression due to myofascial pain, or compression of the nerve by the muscle or tendon with hip internal rotation.

## Risk Factors

- Activities that increase hip external rotation
- Blunt trauma to the gluteal region
- Pregnancy
- Prolonged sitting on hard surfaces

## Clinical Features

- Considered a diagnosis of exclusion
- No consensus on clinical findings
- "Sciaticalike" features

## Natural History

- Progressive limp may overload adjacent structures

## Diagnosis

### *Differential diagnosis*

- Endometriosis
- Herniated nucleus pulposus
- Hip joint pathology
- Pelvic tumors
- Sacroiliac joint pathology
- Spinal stenosis
- Spondylosis

### *History*

- Sitting intolerance
- Buttock pain with or without radiation into the posterior lower extremity
- Pain improves with recumbency and worsens with activity.

### *Exam*

- A limp may develop in the affected side.
- The straight leg raise sign may be positive.
- Pace test increases pain with resisted leg abduction in a sitting position.
- Beatty test places the patient in a side-lying position with the painful side up, the painful leg flexed with the knee resting on the table. Buttock pain develops when the patient holds the knee off the table.
- Freiberg test forcefully rotates the extended thigh internally to elicit buttock pain by stretching the piriformis muscle.
- FADIR test: buttock pain with hip flexion, adduction, and internal rotation
- Palpation may note a characteristic tender palpable mass within the piriformis muscle or the sciatic notch.

### *Testing*

- Bone scan may note an increased uptake.
- Muscle enlargement may be found on MRI or CT.
- Nerve conduction testing demonstrates conduction delays in F waves and H reflexes.

- EMG testing may demonstrate denervation potentials below the piriformis muscle.
- FADIR positioning has been shown to delay the H reflex.

### Pitfalls
- Missed diagnosis

## Red Flags
- Other sacroiliac or hip joint pathology

## Treatment

### Medical
- NSAIDs
- Analgesics
- Muscle relaxants

### Exercises
- Piriformis muscle stretching with internal rotation, hip adduction, and flexion
- Thiele's massage (transrectal massage)

### Modalities
- Heat, cold, ultrasound, and transcutaneous electrical nerve stimulation have been used for symptomatic relief of pain and muscle spasms.

### Injection
- Trigger point injections for symptoms of myofascial pain
- Perisciatic corticosteroid injection
- Caudal epidural steroid injection for radicular symptoms
- Botulinum toxin injection

### Surgical
- Surgical release of the piriformis muscle results in only a minor change in strength in the external rotators and abductors of the hip.

### Consults
- Physical medicine and rehabilitation
- General surgery

### Complications of treatment
- Progressive limp may overload adjacent structures
- Nerve injury related to injections

## Prognosis
- Generally assumed to be good, although small case series have reported good results with surgical release

## Helpful Hints
- The history and physical examination allow the practitioner to exclude other causes in the differential diagnosis.

## Suggested Readings

Fishman LM, Dombi GW, Michaelsen C, et al. Piriformis syndrome: diagnosis, treatment, and outcome, a 10-year study. *Arch Phys Med Rehabil.* 2002;83(3):295–301.

Papadopoulos EC, Khan SN. Piriformis syndrome and low back pain: a new classification and review of the literature. *Orthop Clin North Am.* 2004;35(1):65–67.

# Polymyalgia Rheumatica

## Description

Polymyalgia rheumatica is a clinical syndrome characterized by severe pain and tenderness in the proximal musculature of the extremities.

## Etiology/Types

- Unknown

## Epidemiology

- Incidence is generally 11 per 100,000 individuals.
- Incidence is 50 to 100 cases per 100,000 people in individuals ≥50 years old
- Male to female ratio is 1:4.

## Pathogenesis

- Thought to be an arthritic condition affecting the axial joints.
- Possible immunologic and viral causes

## Risk Factors

- Unknown

## Clinical Features

- Diagnostic criteria include age over 50 years; bilateral neck, shoulder, or pelvic girdle pain; more than 1 hour of morning stiffness; erythrocyte sedimentation rate >40 mm/h; a rapid response to prednisone; and an exclusion of other diagnoses
- Classically found in females over 50 years of age having symmetric neck and shoulder pain and stiffness
- Sternoclavicular and the humeroscapular joints are the most commonly affected joints.
- 70% to 90% describe neck and shoulder pain.
- 50% to 70% describe lower back, pelvic, and thigh pain.
- Pain usually starts in the neck and shoulders and is worse in the morning or with inactivity.
- Constitutional symptoms may be present, such as fever and malaise
- A history of a recent illness may also be noted.

## Natural History

- Usually a benign course that may last from 2 to 4 years

## Diagnosis

### *Differential diagnosis*

- Fibromyalgia
- Giant cell arteritis
- Malignancy
- Myofascial pain syndrome
- Osteoarthritis
- Polymyositis
- Rheumatoid arthritis
- Subacute bacterial endocarditis
- Thyroid or parathyroid dysfunction
- Viral infection

### *History*

- Females over 50 years of age
- History of recent illness
- Pain that is worse in the morning or with inactivity and pain improved with activity
- Diffuse ache in the neck, shoulders, lower back, and pelvic girdle

### *Exam*

- Characteristic muscle tenderness to palpation and activity
- Pain-limited joint active range of motion
- Full-joint passive range of motion
- Possible peripheral asymmetrical arthritis

### *Testing*

- Elevated erythrocyte sedimentation rate
- Occasionally there may also be hypochromic anemia and increased alkaline phosphatase
- Muscle biopsy specimens are normal.
- X-rays are usually unremarkable.
- Bone scan may demonstrate increased uptake in the shoulder joints.
- MRI may demonstrate subacromial or subdeltoid bursitis as well as synovitis of the hip.

### *Pitfalls*

- Missed diagnosis

## Red Flags

- None

## Treatment

### *Medical*

- Daily oral corticosteroids usually improve symptoms within 24 to 48 hours.
- Dose is titrated downward as the patient remains stable.

- NSAIDs may be helpful in pain control for patients with mild disease

### *Exercises*

- General conditioning exercises and range of motion stretching

### *Modalities*

- Heat, cold, ultrasound, and transcutaneous electrical nerve stimulation have been used for symptomatic relief of pain and muscle spasms.

### *Injection*

- Intramuscular methylprednisolone every 3 to 4 weeks has been shown to control symptoms.
- Trigger point injections for symptoms of myofascial pain

### *Surgical*

- None

### *Consults*

- Rheumatology
- Physical medicine and rehabilitation

### *Complications of treatment*

- Related to prolonged corticosteroid use including osteoporosis and immune suppression

## Prognosis

- There is a 30% relapse rate for patients who discontinue oral corticosteroids before 2 years.
- Corticosteroid therapy may continue for 57 years.
- The course of the disease usually lasts from 2 to 4 years.

## Helpful Hints

- Need to exclude other diagnoses
- Benign course

## Suggested Readings

Nothnagl T, Leeb BF. Diagnosis, differential diagnosis and treatment of polymyalgia rheumatica. *Drugs Aging.* 2006;23(5):391–402.

Soubrier M, Dubost JJ, Ristori JM. Polymyalgia rheumatica: diagnosis and treatment. *J Bone Spine.* 2006;73(6):599–605.

# Psychological/Psychiatric Issues

## Description
Psychological barriers to pain resolution

## Etiology/Types
- Somatoform disorders include conversion disorder, somatization disorder, body dismorphic disorder, hypochondriasis, and pain disorder.
- Psychogenic rheumatism includes musculoskeletal complaints in the absence of organic disease and a diagnosed psychiatric illness.
- Camptocormia describes a condition where, following a trivial injury, the individual is bent forward with arms hanging loosely with a downward gaze. Common in industrial workers and soldiers
- Conversion disorder is a syndrome affecting the voluntary nervous system that contraindicates normal musculoskeletal and neurologic physiology,
- Malingering is a conscious misrepresentation of signs and symptoms for secondary gain,

## Epidemiology
- 22% to 66% of psychiatric patients report pain.
- 25% of psychiatric patients report severe pain.
- Lower back is the most common site of pain.
- Other sites of pain include the head, neck, chest, flank, pelvis, and the entire body.
- Malingering is most common in the workplace and is associated with workers' compensation.
- Fewer than 5% of patients with back pain are thought to be malingerers.

## Pathogenesis
- Possibly related to increased anxiety, hysteria, muscle tension, and hallucination

## Risk Factors
- Risk factors for conversion disorders include young females with limited education, low income, and difficulty expressing distress.

## Clinical Features
- Very difficult to differentiate
- Conversion disorder includes loss of extremity function or bowel or bladder dysfunction.

## Natural History
- Variable



## Diagnosis

### *Differential diagnosis*
- Organic versus nonorganic illnesses

### *History*
- Pain drawings demonstrate large areas of pain
- Difficulty with tasks associated with mobility and activities of daily living

### *Exam*
- Conversion disorder demonstrates an inconsistent exam.
- Malingering patients may refuse to participate in components of the exam.
- Normal lumbar or cervical lordosis with no paraspinal muscle spasm is unlikely in a patient with a history of chronic pain.
- Variable tenderness to palpation during the exam
- Intense pain and withdrawal with light palpation
- Hoover's test is done with the patient supine. The examiner places both hands underneath the patient's heels and then asks the patient to raise one leg. Normally, there should be downward pressure on the contralateral heel; if no pressure is noted then malingering may be suspected.
- Cog-wheel rigidity or sudden give-way weakness
- Hyperactive deep tendon reflexes
- Waddell signs include diffuse nonspecific tenderness, overreaction, regionalization, distraction, and stimulation.

### *Testing*
- Imaging studies may be used to rule out significant pathology
- Electrodiagnostic studies may help to differentiate pathology.

### *Pitfalls*
- Overlooked organic illness

## Red Flags
- Neurologic deficits
- Suicidal ideations

## Treatment

### *Medical*
- Psychiatric medications consistent with the psychiatric diagnosis
- Psychotherapy

### Exercises

- Sequential exercise regimens have been used to overcome patient's fear, avoidance, or conversion disorder and return the patient to normal function.
- It may be difficult to convince a patient to participate in an exercise program.

### Modalities

- Heat, cold, ultrasound, and transcutaneous electrical nerve stimulation have been used for symptomatic relief of pain and muscle spasms.

### Injection

- None

### Surgical

- None

### Consults

- Psychiatry
- Psychology
- Physical medicine and rehabilitation
- Referral to another physician for a second unbiased opinion

### Complications of treatment

- Variable

## Prognosis

- 60% of conversion disorders may improve within 2 weeks; 98% will improve in one year with identification of underlying stress and normal findings
- 25% of conversion disorder patients have recurrence within the first year.
- Some patients with spinal pain may not improve.

## Helpful Hints

- Always be alert for a possible organic illness

## Suggested Readings

Letonoff EJ, Williams TR, Sidhu KS. Hysterical paralysis: a report of three cases and a review of the literature. *Spine.* 2002;27(20):E441–E445.

McDermott BE, Feldman MD. Malingering in the medical setting. *Psychiatr Clin North Am.* 2007;30(4):645–662.

Rashbaum IG, Sarno JE. Psychosomatic concepts in chronic pain. *Arch Phys Med Rehabil.* 2003;84(3 suppl 1): S76–S80.

Trieschmann RB, Stolov WC, Montgomery ED. An approach to the treatment of abnormal ambulation resulting from conversion reaction. *Arch Phys Med Rehabil.* 1970;51(4):198–206.

# Shoulder Impingement Syndrome

## Description

Shoulder impingement syndrome is the most common disorder of the shoulder.

## Etiology/Types

- Subacromial bursitis, partial rotator cuff tears, rotator cuff tendinosis, and calcified tendonitis

## Epidemiology

- Incidence of shoulder pathology ranges from 7 to 25 per 1,000 visits to primary care physicians.
- Prevalence ranges from 7% to 27% in those <70 years of age and 13% to 26% in those >70 years of age.

## Pathogenesis

- Repetitive or excessive contact or abrasion of the rotator cuff muscles and/or tendons due to compression between the humeral head and acromion, coracoacromial ligament, and acromioclavicular joint.

## Risk Factors

- Deconditioning
- Neurologic injuries
- Sports involving throwing or overhead activities
- Trauma

## Clinical Features

- Shoulder pain causes pain along the scapula and trapezius muscle, but not the neck; pain worsens with forward flexion of the shoulder; pain is often referred to the lateral shoulder and mid-arm. Patients note difficultly in removing a shirt or coat.
- Cervical pathology can radiate into the shoulder and shoulder pathology can radiate into the neck.
- Cervical pathology may lead to secondary shoulder disease, such as frozen shoulder.
- Atrophy of the shoulder musculature can be associated with either C5 or C6 radiculopathy or chronic rotator cuff injury.
- Active shoulder range of motion limitations may be related to deltoid or rotator cuff weakness, resulting from a cervical radiculopathy or disuse atrophy caused by pain.

## Natural History

- Progresses from edema and hemorrhage to cuff fibrosis and thickening or a partial cuff tear and finally develops into full thickness tears, tendon ruptures, and bony changes.

## Diagnosis

### *Differential diagnosis*

- Cervical disc herniation with radiculopathy
- Cervical myelopathy
- Cervical spondylosis
- Frozen shoulder
- Glenohumeral instability or osteoarthritis
- Lung tumors
- Nerve palsies
- Shoulder impingement syndrome

### *History*

- Pain with shoulder range of motion
- Difficulty or pain with putting on shirts or coats
- Difficulty or pain with overhead activities
- Pain at night
- Pain located deep in the shoulder or in the lateral proximal arm

### *Exam*

- Inspection of muscle tone, symmetry, and deformity
- Palpation to assess for areas of swelling, tenderness or other abnormalities
- Active and passive neck and shoulder range of motion
- Strength testing of the upper extremities
- Biceps, triceps, and brachioradialis reflex testing
- Sensation testing of the upper extremities
- Neer's and Hawkin's impingement signs
- Resisted abduction of the arm tests strength and may also reproduce pain
- The best combination for subacromial impingement syndrome are the Hawkins sign, external rotation weakness, and horizontal abduction

### *Testing*

- X-rays of the shoulder should include anterior–posterior, lateral, and axillary views
- MRI is the study of choice for assessing for rotator cuff tears.
- MRI may detect rotator cuff tears in 34% of asymptomatic individuals and this frequency increases with age
- CT is useful in diagnosing subtle dislocations, labral tears, full thickness rotator cuff tears, bony lesions, or subtle dislocation.

- Musculoskeletal ultrasonography
- Electrodiagnostic studies are useful in differentiating shoulder pathology from radiculopathy and myopathy as well as determining the severity and chronicity of the neurologic process.

### *Pitfalls*

- MRI findings may not correlate with the patient's symptoms

## Red Flags

- Joint infection
- Fracture
- Glenohumeral dislocation

## Treatment

### *Medical*

- Rest
- Ice
- NSAIDs
- Acetaminophen

### *Exercises*

- Progressive strengthening exercises of the rotator cuff muscles

### *Modalities*

- Heat, cold, ultrasound, and transcutaneous electrical nerve stimulation have been used for symptomatic relief of pain and muscle spasms.

### *Injection*

- Anesthetic injection into the subacromial region can help with diagnosis and treatment.
- Intra-articular or subacromial corticosteroid and anesthetic injections have been shown to provide short-term relief.
- Intra-articular sodium hyaluronates into the glenohumeral joint or bursa have been well tolerated.
- Intra-articular injections should be done under imaging guidance, if available.

### *Surgical*

- Open acromioplasty and rotator cuff repair in 21 patients with electrodiagnostically documented cervical radiculopathy has demonstrated decreased shoulder pain in 87% of patients and decreased neck pain in 66% of patients.

### *Consults*

- Physical medicine and rehabilitation
- Orthopedic surgery

### *Complications of treatment*

- Complications related to surgery

## Prognosis

- Progression of a partial rotator cuff tear to a full tear with loss of shoulder function
- Mobility may be maintained even with evidence of a full rotator cuff tear.

## Helpful Hints

- Emphasis on strengthening and stretching

## Suggested Reading

Hawkins RJ, Bilco T, Bonutti P. Cervical spine and shoulder pain. *Clin Orthop Relat Res.* 1990;(258):142–146.

# Trochanteric Bursitis

## Description

Trochanteric bursitis is a regional pain syndrome described as an aching intermittent pain over the lateral hip region.

## Etiology/Types

- Acute, subacute, and chronic types

## Epidemiology

- One of the most common causes of hip pain
- Incidence is 1.8 to 5.6 per 1,000 adults in 1 year
- Most common in the 40- to 60-year-old age group, but found in all age groups
- Female to male ratio is of 2–4:1.

## Pathogenesis

- Gluteus minimus bursa lies slightly anterior and above the proximal superior surface of the greater trochanter.
- Subgluteus medius bursa lies underneath the gluteus medius muscle and is located supra-posteriorly of the proximal edge of the greater trochanter.
- Subgluteus maximus bursa is 4 to 6 cm long and 24 cm wide and located lateral to the greater trochanter at the convergence of the tensor fascia lata and gluteus maximus, as they form the iliotibial tract.
  - Allows the anterior part of the gluteus maximus tendon to pass over the trochanter to insert into the iliotibial band.
  - Irritation results in trochanteric bursitis.

## Risk Factors

- Biomechanical alterations in the lower extremity such as lower-extremity joint osteoarthritis
- Tendinous calcification
- Deconditioning
- Degenerative hip changes
- Hemiparesis
- Iliotibial band syndrome
- Leg-length discrepancy
- Lumbar spondylosis
- Obesity
- Pes planus
- Radiculopathy
- Repetitive microtrauma
- Residual weakness following spine or hip surgery
- Total hip arthroplasty
- Trauma is noted in up to 64% of patients.

## Clinical Features

- Acute, subacute, or chronic intermittent sharp or aching pain on the lateral hip
- Radiation into the lateral thigh occurs in 25% to 40% of cases.
- Maximal tenderness is often at the junction of the upper thigh and greater trochanter.
- Maximal tenderness can be located just posterior to the apex of the greater trochanter.
- Most often worsened with active hip external rotation and abduction
- Occasionally worsens with active internal rotation or extension of the hip
- Worsens with prolonged standing, prolonged walking, running, and ascending or descending stairs

## Natural History

- May lead to calcification in the region of the greater trochanter
- May lead to significant disability
- May last months to years
- Some clinicians believe it is a self-limiting disease.

## Diagnosis

### *Differential diagnosis*

- Acetabular labral tear
- Avascular necrosis
- Femoral neck stress fracture
- Gluteus minimus and medius tears or tendonitis
- Hip osteoarthritis
- Lumbar compression fractures
- Lumbar spine degenerative changes
- Lumbar radiculopathy

### *History*

- Waxing and waning pain
- Lateral hip pain that radiates down the lateral thigh but rarely to the knee or below.
- Worsens with climbing stairs, sleeping on the ipsilateral side, or at night in general

### *Exam*

- Palpation of the greater trochanter at the insertion of the gluteus medius muscle

- "Jump" sign at the site of maximal tenderness on the greater trochanter
- Positive FABER test

### Testing
- X-rays may demonstrate calcifications in the region of the greater trochanter and an irregular surface of the greater trochanter
- MRI may demonstrate increased signal on short tau inversion recovery sequences and distension of the greater trochanteric bursa.
- Bone scan may demonstrate increased uptake in the region of the greater trochanter
- Musculoskeletal ultrasound may demonstrate enlargement of the subgluteus maximus bursa, deep trochanteric bursa of the gluteus medius, and minimus.

### Pitfalls
- Trochanteric bursitis is found in 18% to 45% of patients who present with low back pain.
- Pseudoradiculopathy that presents with radiation of pain along the iliotibial tract mimics nerve root irritation.

## Red Flags
- Hip fracture

## Treatment

### Medical
- Behavior modification
- Weight loss
- NSAIDs
- Contralateral heel lift for leg-length discrepancy
- Use of a cane

### Exercises
- Hip and lower back strengthening and stretching

### Modalities
- Heat, cold, ultrasound, and transcutaneous electrical nerve stimulation have been used for symptomatic relief of pain and muscle spasms.

### Injection
- Blind corticosteroid and anesthetic injections at the site of maximal tenderness with surrounding infiltration
- Musculoskeletal ultrasound and fluoroscopic guidance have been used to more accurately target the bursae with improved outcomes.

### Surgical
- Considered in refractory cases
- Considered for excision of the calcifications, bursal sac, and iliotibial band release with good results in small case series

### Consults
- Physical medicine and rehabilitation
- Orthopedic surgery

### Complications of treatment
- Complications related to surgery

## Prognosis
- Depending on the underlying etiology may last for years

## Helpful Hints
- Trochanteric bursitis may be a primary or secondary diagnosis in patients with low back pain

## Suggested Reading
Shbeeb MI, Matteson EL.Trochanteric bursitis (greater trochanter pain syndrome). *Mayo Clin Proc.* 1996;71(6):565–569.

# Index